TOUGH LOVE *Letters*

LIFE CHANGING SECRETS
for the FAT, UNFIT, UNHEALTHY, *and* UNHAPPY

....

ALBERT EILER

Illustrated by Sophia Marie Pappas

D1512334

Facilitated by Sue Seiff

Illustrations by Sophia Marie Pappas

Edited by Beth Wojiski

Cover and interior designed by Stewart Williams

ISBN: 978-1701621176

www.alltrainllc.com
www.alltrainllc.com/plain
www.aerights.com
www.agewellllc.com

For my girls...you embolden me.

"If you don't like your life...change it."
~Anonymous

CONTENTS

Acknowledgments

I'm beyond grateful to Sue Seiff for facilitating this project. Your skill set is crazy diverse, your work ethic is second to none, and what you don't know today you always know tomorrow. Thank you for listening, thank you for believing, thank you for bantering, thank you for challenging me, thank you for the precious time you've sacrificed to work on my "butterfly" concepts...and thank you for making me laugh over the years—all nine times. Now get out of my head; there's room for only one demented mind in here!

Thank you to Sophia Pappas for your creatively animated illustrations. Your talent is remarkable, and your innate ability to capture the traits we requested in an illustration is extraordinary. It's ironic that we connected through the familiarity of my hometown zip code...go North Side!

Thank you to Beth Wojiski for editing away on this project. Your expertise, efficiency, and willingness to always fit this project in are greatly appreciated. Your knowledge of the use of the ellipses is deep :) and your appreciation of an iconic muscle car is impressive...you gearhead!

Thank you to Stewart Williams for your clever vision in the design of this initiative. Your patience in hearing me out not once, not twice, but three times is greatly appreciated, as I know I infringed a touch on those off-the-grid bike rides you rightfully cherish. And man, who knew you're right here in the 'Burgh climbing the same hills I grew up training on myself.

A very special thank you to my badass Beta Read Team. I greatly appreciate you taking the time to review the manuscript and your willingness to approach me with your feedback, opinions, and constructive criticism. Note, however: if this book gets bad reviews, it's all your fault.

Finally, I thank the thousands of clients and prospects I have worked or consulted with over the past 25 years. Thank you for taking the initiative to improved well-being. Without our interactions, my coaching career could not have been a success, and this project would not be possible.

Foreword

Throughout my professional life, I have read thousands of op-eds, listened to countless talk show pundits, and endured the legislative foolishness of self-acclaimed healthcare experts. I have anxiously awaited someone to emerge and deliver the kind of gut-punching messages reflected in Albert Eiler's *Tough Love Letters*. Bravo. The simplicity in Eiler's revelations is a thing of beauty.

While it's clear this life manual spawned from the tenacious passion oozing from the author's vast experience in personal training, life coaching, and wellness programming, as a physician I can't overlook its relevance in today's healthcare climate. Primarily, that **Wellness**—making lifestyle choices that promote long-term health and strive to prevent injury and disease—is the salient key to cutting costs. **Wellness** is the ultimate answer to solving the access problem. **Wellness** shifts the responsibility for quality of life from the provider to the patient.

Recognizing the blatantly clear connection Eiler makes between behavior and wellness, I am grateful for this opportunity to preface this book and its colloquial storytelling with my own perspective from the trenches of patient care. My specialty in Orthopaedics exposes me to daily interactions with people of all ages and walks of life. It saddens me to encounter so many folks who are utterly dazed and confused when it comes to taking care of themselves.

I'm dumbfounded by the number of young people who lack a primary care physician to oversee the stages of life and focus on disease prevention. Some request to directly see specialists for paper cuts, splinters, or three days of elbow pain.

Fortysomethings carry excess weight on their joints for years and then curse insurance companies for setting stricter criteria to approve having those joints replaced with imperfect and unnatural metal and plastic parts. Bullheaded retirees cling to ill-conceived medical recommendations from neighbors, golfing buddies, and other acquaintances, rather than educate themselves or heed the advice of trained professionals. A few wait until their carpal tunnel syndrome is irreversible and then expect a miraculous reversal of permanent nerve damage by the assumed panacea of surgical intervention.

Ironically, it wouldn't take long to collect a similar series of patient foibles from my clinic to reinforce what is so blatantly and devastatingly going wrong with the average Joe.

After feasting on the morsels of wisdom throughout this book, several major themes resonated in the context of the American healthcare system. If a real metamorphosis is desired, let these tenets that I've gleaned from the pages of Eiler's *Tough Love Letters* guide us:

1. Take the best care of yourself that you can through proper nutrition and exercise.
2. Make well-being a responsibility, and don't expect others to do it for you (nor carry the burden for it if you don't).

3. Budget for unforeseen health problems before consuming the luxuries of life.
4. Lead your offspring, dependents, and employees (if you have them) by example.
5. Figure out how you can make your time on this earth matter to those who truly matter to you.

What is artfully presented within the pages of *Tough Love Letters* supersedes decades upon decades of hackneyed publications on wellness—ranging from the ostentatiously scientific to the deceitfully exploitative to the unequivocally erroneous—through 25 real-life vignettes and the justifiable smackdowns that follow. One after another, Albert Eiler delivers 95 mph four-seamers and dares us to connect with transformational exit velocity. Beneath the harsh veneer is the kind of no-nonsense sincerity so often missing in our everyday dialogue and so desperately necessary to inculcate the youth of this "softening" (both physically and emotionally) nation.

Lance M. Brunton, MD
Excela Health Orthopaedics and Sports Medicine
Latrobe, Pennsylvania

About the Author

Albert Eiler is a tough-love truth teller who guides those seeking a leaner, healthier, higher-performing, and happier life by tapping into his experience as an entrepreneur, fitness and performance trainer, nutrition realist, author, gentleman farmer, youth sports coach, husband, and father to two lovely and lively daughters. He has spent over 25 years in the fitness and wellness industry, and has observed firsthand much **deceit** (i.e., the quick-fix, fountain-of-youth marketing ploys of many supplement distributors, equipment manufacturers, and fitness franchises), **desperation** (i.e., folks taking foolhardy and risky measures), and **disillusion** (i.e., many engaging in irrational, ill-fated health experiments.)

In 1997, at age 27, Eiler opened his own performance, fitness, and nutrition training center, a 9000-square-foot facility where he and his group of coaches trained recreational, high school, collegiate, and professional athletes, working professionals, and cool stay-at-home moms and dads. Eight years later he established ChangeRx, a nationally reaching corporate wellness company deeply rooted in education. In 2017, he founded **ALLTRAIN** and **PLAIN**— brands that have enabled him to deliver his core principles of training and nutrition to a much broader audience. And in 2019 he launched AErights.com, where a collection of his writings on physical performance, nutrition, youth sports, and parenting, as well as children's stories, reside.

Early on in his career, he chose to stray from the norm of so many health clubs, high-intensity class-based gyms, corporate wellness firms, coaches, and self-proclaimed fitness gurus who offered quick or dicey fixes to the vulnerable masses. His commitment to coaching and educating his clients in strategic, safe, and sustainable training and nutrition continues to this day.

Eiler practices what he preaches. As he navigates life in his late forties, he implements his training plans to stay strong and supple while avoiding injury, produces much of his own food through fishing, farming, and foraging (well, except for pizza-and-ice-cream Sundays with his family), and has kept his business aspirations in check to spend more time with his three "gals."

To learn more and find Albert Eiler's resources online:
alltrainllc.com
alltrainllc.com/plain
aerights.com
agewellllc.com

Tough Love Welcome

Since you've picked up *Tough Love Letters, Life Changing Secrets for the Fat, Unfit, Unhealthy...and Unhappy*, you're likely looking for a solution to your own or a loved one's struggles...or maybe you're just intrigued by the title.

In any case, I'm stoked[1] to have you aboard.

I think this book has been writing itself in the back of my slightly demented, yet what I've been told is my "oddly observant" mind since the day my wellness career began over 25 years ago. I observe behavior, and at the risk of sounding cliché and slightly alliteration-crazy: people and their plights are my passion.

The idea of penning a regular old diet and exercise how-to book has never excited me. Throughout my coaching career and in my writings, I've tried to dig deeper into the why: why she struggles, why he struggles, why real people do really stupid things when it comes to their overall well-being. However, writing a book about real people I've known seemed like a less-than-stellar idea. So instead, the 25 crazed and confused characters I've brought to life on these pages each represents a composite of many well-meaning but misguided people I've encountered or observed in my roles as a trainer, sports performance coach,

---

[1] I've always wanted to use the word "stoked" in an effort to portray myself as cool.

wellness consultant, nutrition realist, and business owner.

Collectively, my 25 characters are a reflection of a large (pun intended) majority of our society that depicts:

- **The Fat:** (yes, I used the "F-word"): While it's not pleasant to hear (or write), it's reality. Overweight and obese frames carry excess body fat that often causes lack of confidence, recurring embarrassment, extreme fatigue, restricted movement, orthopedic injuries, and countless other health issues;
- **The Unfit:** Of course, those who don't make exercise (or what I prefer to call "training") a priority in their lives tend to be unfit. But in *Tough Love Letters*, I'm also labeling those who train in such a way that they create injury-laden, dysfunctional bodies (some that may even appear fit but in reality are not) as unfit;
- **The Unhealthy:** By that I don't just mean the physically unhealthy, with issues such as elevated blood pressure, high cholesterol, prediabetes, and sleep apnea that are often self-inflicted through poor lifestyle behaviors. So many of my characters also possess an unhealthy obsession with wealth, material goods, social media, food, and the idolization of sports figures and celebrities; and
- **The Unhappy:** Well, basically all of my characters are unhappy—that's why they're in the book.

While each character possesses a different "feature flaw" as his or her name may suggest, most of them share a common reality: an unsatisfying, dysfunctional life that has spiraled out of control. Many have created overbooked, overworked, overstimulated, chronically stressed, and in some respects unpurposeful lives. Their daily obsessions with money, possessions, gluttonous food conquests, and the desire to live life through others are wreaking havoc on their body composition, general health, fitness, physical and mental performance, and happiness.

To make matters worse, they make naive attempts at transformation that are quite often just plain nonsense—where they open Pandora's box of perilous paths—experiencing very little results aside from short term. Some are duped by the fitness industry's marketing monster of 24/7 fitness centers at a cost of pennies per day. And others are led to believe that high-intensity group training will bring back the fountain of youth. Countless others look to superfood smoothies, seaweed detoxes, and the like to turn back time.

In a nutshell, these characters were brought to life with a clear and revealing purpose in mind. As you read the chapters—one for each character—see if you identify with one or more of them. Are you a Low-Carb Larry? A Detox Debbie? An All-Business Alison? Maybe a Marathon Marvin or a Fitness-Freak Faith? Or perhaps you and your family are living the same life as Travel-Ball Tammy and her family? Keep in mind that while you may not relate "directly" to a specific character, there likely will be a few traits that you will "indirectly" relate to within each chapter. And by becoming acquainted with these characters' lives, you will soon begin to see that so many of us deal with eerily similar struggles. Their struggles, your struggles, and mine—yeah, I'm not remotely perfect—are so often the result of our own choices, laziness, need, and greed.

Still with me?

If so, remain calm, and continue on. At the end of each

chapter, I've written my character a tough love letter filled with clear-cut calls to action that might be painful to hear but are honest, highly effective, and based on my insight from real-life experience.

With nearly three decades spent helping countless clients realize true well-being, I've written this book not to throw stones or judge. Instead, it is my sincere hope that *Tough Love Letters* will serve as an eye- and mind-opening guide for many more folks who are fat, physically unfit, financially stressed, floundering when it comes to their health, frustrated with failed attempts at change, or feeling lost and unhappy.

I ask this favor: please put aside any preconceived notions or boiling tempers that may arise from this read. Embrace the message with a receptive mind. Grasp humility tightly, and take a big step toward transformation.

Albert Eiler ("AE")

Cast of Characters

Detox Debbie

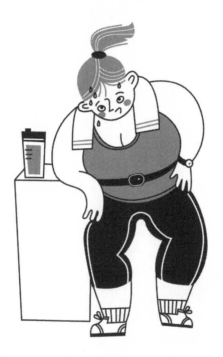

D ebbie is in her late 30s and has struggled with her weight since her first year of college. She got hit with the "freshman fifteen" and then some and has been battling a roller coaster of weight gain and weight loss for close to 20 years. At 5'2", Debbie currently weighs 175 pounds with a body fat percentage of 44 percent, which means she carries 77 pounds of fat!

Debbie is obsessed with her weight. She attends The Pulse Zone, a gym where she spends most of her hour-long class focused on her cardio, specifically on the rower and bike, and where a mic'd, quasi-cheerleading trainer pushes her and her classmates to "stay in the zone." Debbie frequently glances up at the progress screen to make sure her heart rate, which is monitored by a device strapped around her chest, is optimized (in the "Pulse Zone") and that she burns at least 500 calories by the end of the class.

The Pulse Zone, a cardio-focused chain gym with its month-by-month membership option, works well for Debbie because she generally commits herself back to an exercise regimen when she's simultaneously decided to "detox" again.

Debbie's detox days began in her late 20s when she met a nutrition guru named Dr. Dean. Debbie had heard about Dean from some of her coworkers, who referred to him as a "holistic expert" who had a special "detoxification" formula that was helping so many people lose weight. While already in the midst of her weight struggle, Debbie was willing to try anything.

So Debbie set up an appointment with Dean at his chiropractic office. After an initial, two-hour complimentary consultation where she and Dean discussed her struggles and reviewed testimonial after testimonial from Dean's clients, Debbie agreed to an extensive blood panel profile based on his strong recommendation. Though quite expensive at a cost of $700.00 and unfortunately not covered under her health plan, Debbie trusted Dean, and in her mind, his success stories alone were enough to win her over.

Within a week, Debbie was called in to review her results with Dean (this time costing $175 for an office visit), and Debbie discovered she had numerous deficiencies and allergies (many of which she could not pronounce) that affected her ability to lose weight. But she was so relieved to learn that there were reasons behind her struggles, and even more so, that there were solutions. Debbie agreed with Dean's suggestions for a detox and supplementation program, bought her first month's worth right on the spot, and signed up for the formulas to be sent directly to her house moving forward each month at a cost of $199 per month. The monthly fee would be conveniently deducted from her checking account via monthly debit.

The very next day, Debbie was mixing and consuming her seaweed-green, ingredient-rich, fiber-filled shakes three times per day, joined a gym, and began performing her cardio-heavy workouts five days a week—and spent quite a bit of time on the toilet.

After just one week, she dropped ten pounds! She was absolutely tickled with herself! Furthermore, at her three-week follow-up with Dean (and another $175 office visit), she was down a total of 18 pounds! Debbie had never experienced this kind of rapid weight loss in her life.

Debbie was on cloud nine. After seven weeks, she was down 35 pounds, and even better, she began dating a great guy named Derek, whom she met at The Pulse Zone.

With the fling and newfound motivation, Debbie added another visit with Dr. Dean. With this extra visit came additional vitamins, a proprietary formulated bar for when Debbie could start eating whole foods, and special drops designed to suppress her appetite. (Note: the monthly debit to her checking account was up to $279, but she felt she was well worth it.)

Unfortunately Debbie's happy streak came to a

screeching halt at Week 10. Just a month into her hot and heavy relationship with Derek, she found out she was not the only woman he was dating at The Pulse Zone. Debbie dumped Derek and found herself distraught. She went back to familiar ways: finding comfort in food and spending much of her free time at home snuggling up with a blanket in front of the TV with cookies, chips, and hot cocoa. When she did make it out, it was to meet a couple of girlfriends at her neighborhood pub, where she had a few drinks and appetizers and talked about her breakup. Debbie also gave up the gym, as she just couldn't drag herself there.

Within four weeks of self-pity, Debbie has gained all of her weight back, as well as an additional five pounds. She couldn't believe this had happened! Less than two months ago she was at the top of her game. But after three more weeks went by and another four pounds went on, Debbie knew it was time to recommit herself. Her bank account was still being hit with those monthly automatic charges for the detox program, and she had two months' worth of detox formula in her cupboard already. So the detox cycle began again. She started down the path that enabled her to lose the weight so quickly the first time. Green shakes three times per day, a bunch of cardio, and of course a lot of time in the bathroom. And while the weight wasn't dropping as quickly as she would like, Debbie had managed to drop 14 pounds in four weeks.

However, Debbie was still feeling lonely and she desperately wanted to be social, so she accepted an invitation for a girls' night out. At the bar, she slipped up and had a few drinks, which caused her to drop her guard. She ended up consuming quite a bit of rich, high-calorie, solid foods that she hadn't touched in over a month. The taste was almost insatiable, and on her way home she couldn't help but stop and grab some late-night pastries for a bedtime snack. She awoke the next morning to feelings of guilt and shame for acting so out of control the night before. In an attempt to offset her evening of gluttony, she hit the gym for a two-hour cardio fest and skipped two of her green shakes—less is more, right? But the next day, her urges got the best of her and she found herself at the grocery store bakery aisle buying everything in sight.

Off she went on another roller coaster ride of weight gain, until her next attempt at a "detox."

To this day she continues her weight losses and gains, each time returning to her old ways: attacking her weight with what she thought "worked before."

Dear Debbie,

Stop the cycle of misguided mayhem! You need to look at what has happened to your body composition level over the years. Remember when you lost a lot of weight very rapidly in your very first detoxification? It's highly likely that you lost not only fat weight (note: metabolically inactive weight), but most likely you lost a good bit of precious lean muscle weight (note: metabolically active weight) as well. So even though you were lighter, your metabolism was slower.

When you inevitably broke down from this restrictive plan and went back to eating whole foods (and plenty of unfavorable ones), you gained your weight back and then some, but likely very little of that was muscle. This problem was exaggerated because your workouts consisted primarily of cardio exercises and no significant strength training. You then turned to another "detox" and rapid weight loss, which again likely involved losing some fat and a good bit more muscle, each time gaining back your weight and then some (but with less and less muscle each time). Now you're 45 pounds heavier than you were when you entered college, and from a metabolic standpoint, your fire is barely lit.

Debbie, you need to wake up and recognize the "detox" and excessive cardio quick-fix pattern you've been performing for the past 15 years is in large part the reason for your current condition.

Stop the cycle of misguided mayhem!

Yes, this is probably very disheartening to hear, thinking you've wasted 15 years of time when you thought you were improving your well-being.

But my dear, there is hope, and you have a full life ahead of you. You can turn this around, and within a year that 45 pounds can be long gone and that lean body you so desperately long for can be yours. You need to begin a properly designed training program that will help you increase lean mass and hence your metabolism. You need to begin eating whole, nutrient-rich, nonprocessed foods in a plain and simple fashion.

There are no true quick fixes or magic liquid elixirs. Debbie, forgo the excess chemicals; embrace Mother Nature.

AE

CHAPTER 2

Low-Carb Larry

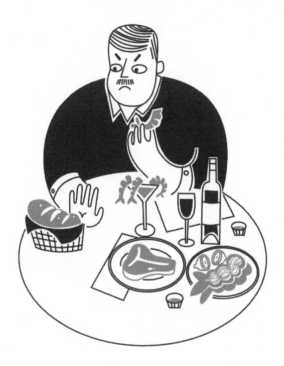

L arry is a 48-year-old, second-generation owner of multiple storage unit complexes across his town, as well as in a few neighboring states. Over the last five years since taking charge of the business, Larry has developed into quite the business man, learning the nuances of this tough but very lucrative business from his father. In fact, Larry has begun to grow the family business substantially, negotiating deals to buy up smaller mom-and-pop shops and developing new state-of-the-art storage units from the ground up.

Managing and negotiating these deals has Larry traveling most days of the week, which inevitably leads him down the road of almost constant entertaining as he's closing deals.

Larry is the father of three teenage children and is married to Lisa, who has been a part-time exercise and physiology professor since leaving her full-time position after the birth of their first child. Larry has fought an excess amount of body fat for most of his adult life, reaching his current state where he sits with a body fat percentage of upward of 35 percent on a 230-pound frame at 5'9" tall. His current physique is a far cry from his high school graduation weight of a much leaner 167 pounds. For all the success Larry has in the business world, he desperately wants to lose weight for his upcoming 20th wedding anniversary, as this 81 pounds of fat that sit on his frame weigh on him heavily.

Ironically, Lisa manages to maintain the same lean weight she was when they married, as she is a big fan of taking care of herself through proper training and eating a variety of nutrient-rich foods prepared, for the most part, in a plain and simple fashion. And she does her absolute best to make sure their children follow these same principles, preparing them healthy meals for breakfast and dinner as well as packing them nutritious lunches for school. In addition, Lisa always has fruits, precut veggies, nuts, and seeds available for quick snacks as she's frequently shuttling them to their school sports practices and games. (It's worth noting that Larry is rarely at home to eat with the family or attend their sporting events.)

Larry knows his body is a mess and wants to look good for his wife on their anniversary trip to the islands. So he's going back to his tried-and-true method of drastically cutting his carbohydrate intake as he always does when he's got a new goal.

Hence, Larry declares war on carbohydrates, cutting out what he believes to be the culprit in his massive fat gain— foods like rice, potatoes, yams, legumes, lentils, bananas, raisins, carrots, snow peas, and pastas and breads as well.

He'll plan to eat large amounts of proteins and fats, where his body will be forced to burn stored body fat for energy rather than the excessive carbohydrates. Larry is a pro at this method. After all, he follows multiple low-carb online forums, and has dropped 20–25 pounds time and time again.

Larry shoots out of the gate as he always does during the first week of his newly dedicated life: with pure determination as he shares with anyone who will listen, including his personal trainer, his employees, and those he's entertaining, about how his method is the ultimate fat-loss technique. He shares podcasts and links to low-carb "gurus" to all of his friends and does his best to get them to join him on his latest carb-cutting quest.

To boost his results, he jumps on his own high-end stationary bike every morning, dialing into his premium account of online, beautifully built instructors with headsets to lead him through his grueling bike ride.

Larry notices the weight dropping quickly during the first week, as he often does, and when he's out entertaining, he hides none of his intentions as he orders finer foods such as high-protein lobster tails loaded with mounds of butter and an iceberg (low in carbs, high in water) wedge salad loaded with blue cheese dressing, blue cheese clumps, and bacon bits, all the while being sure to stay away from the evil, carbohydrate-rich breads that are placed on the table as well as any corn, rice, or potatoes.

Midway through his first week, Larry attacks the grocery store with the same familiar conviction of his past, where he loads up on $30/pound ahi tuna fillets and $20/pound grass-fed steaks, and he hits the bulk nut area for freshly ground almond butter, peanut butter, and cashew butter, as well as a huge container of flaxseeds. He also tags the prepared food section and loads up on guacamole and deviled eggs, and is sure to stock up on a bunch of scrumptious bacon and sausage from the deli section. And last, he grabs low-carb protein bars by the case, making sure he gets his double-chocolate and cookies-and-cream favorites.

Larry's riding high, and after a week of success by way of a 10-pound drop, he figures it's okay to add in a glass or two of red wine after his first week of absolute sacrifice. But he continues to stick to only the finer meats such as Kobe beef with heavy cream, buttered Dover sole, shrimp scampi soaked in margarine, and fried calamari. And he generally finishes dinner with an antipasto plate loaded with cheese, salami, and capicola. Just absolutely no carbohydrate-rich breads, pastas, potatoes, or rice, as they are the enemy. At home he starts to snack on piles of guacamole, nut butters, and deviled eggs, and when he's traveling in his car he's begun to add a few of those low-carb protein bars to hold him over.

Larry's second week is a little less successful, only dropping two pounds, but he's down a total of 12 pounds and feels great!

By the third week, Larry begins to prepare low-carb breakfasts at home, such as four thick slices of bacon, three sausage links, two fried eggs, and a few large tablespoons of nut butter. For lunches out he'll generally order two bacon burgers with no buns and globs of mayo, the low-carb protein bars are up to three or four a day, and the "couple of glasses" of wine are now up to close to a bottle each night.

After the third week, Larry has lost no additional weight and actually has put three pounds back on. He figures the added weight is a result of something salty he ate, so he continues on with his current habits, and also ups his activity on the bike as he realizes he's only biked two times the last two weeks.

Before you know it, Larry and his wife are off to the islands to celebrate, where Larry sits at 221 pounds. By the end of their four-day getaway (and once Larry let his guard down from his ever-so-disciplined low-carb lifestyle), he comes home at his familiar 230-pound mark. Once again he's miserable, as his highly intoxicated state could not mask the embarrassment of how he looked like a balloon sitting on the beach and how he literally floated in the surf.

In true fashion, Larry begins the low-carb approach once again, assuring himself it's "the way" to the physique he so desperately desires.

Dear Larry,

If you want to take the lower-carb approach then you really need to consider proceeding with caution, common sense, and a touch of humility. First, loads of margarine, bacon, sausage, and fried foods? Are you planning out your own demise?

Second, why the need for $30/pound sashimi-grade ahi tuna, Kobe beef with heavy cream, and lobster with mounds of butter at every turn? What's wrong with basic lean meats prepared in a plain and simple fashion? Why not an occasional can of tuna on top of a bed of low-carb but nutrient-rich greens, a basic lean beef patty grilled with nothing but a touch of oil and herbs, then served with steamed mushrooms, peppers and onions, or a simple shrimp cocktail with a low-carb spinach wrap?

Third, why the prepared guacamole and deviled eggs and not just a nice chunk of avocado along with a hard-boiled egg?

Fourth, the freshly ground nut butters at eight bucks a container? Is that really that much "healthier" than bottled natural nut butters at more than half the cost?

Fifth, the low-carb protein bars, Larry? Come on, man. They are nothing but glorified candy bars!

...loads of margarine, bacon, sausage, and fried foods? Are you planning out your own demise?

And finally, the addition of the fancy wines after a week because it's "healthy" and you've earned it based on your one week's "massive" sacrifice of cutting out all other carbs?

Larry, you're acting like an uneducated and spoiled "meat" head—sabotaging your low-carb approach with ignorance and arrogance. Your gluttonous lifestyle while you're out making deals, as well as your rationalizations of what you purchase and consume from your grocery store expeditions, are the reasons you are fat.

Look, Larry, plain steamed rice, baked yams, and boiled pinto beans did not get you into your predicament of 81 pounds of fat on your 230-pound frame. But if low-carb is your gig, you still have to respect Mother Nature and consume foods that can be fished, grown, and butchered and prepared plainly and simply. And for goodness' sake man, add in some micronutrient-rich vegetables like broccoli, kale, and Brussels sprouts and fruits like berries and apples. Larry, the freaking apple and steamed kale didn't turn you into a fat mess.

And bike riding only, Larry? This cardio-only fitness approach is going to do little in the way of adding strength and quality lean mass, nor much in the way of the areas of power development and mobility. You need a well-programmed, comprehensive program.

And last, consider reflecting a little on your pattern of always going back to this "tried-and-true" method of weight loss. The fact you go back to this approach time and again screams there may be something wrong with this picture.

AE

....

CHAPTER 3

Enabling-Parent Pat

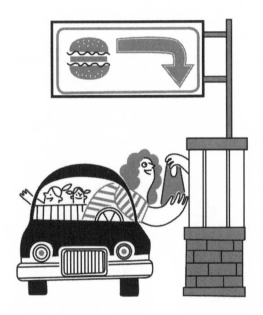

P atrick (a.k.a. "Pat") and Patricia (a.k.a. "Pat") met in grad school, and aside from the obvious, had a bunch of things in common. Both were family-oriented, loved kids, and were each working toward a master's degree in education. And they were athletes. Patrick started playing soccer at age 8 and continued through high school, where he was rather successful, lettering in the sport his junior and senior seasons. Patricia was on the softball field almost as soon as she was out of diapers, and transitioned to lacrosse in high school, where she was selected to the All-Section team as a junior and senior.

"The Pats," as their friends called the cute couple, also played recreational, coed softball, which is how they met. Their budding romance blossomed at their favorite post-game sports bar, Paddy O's. Over appetizers and beer, the young, spirited grad students would map out their future plans for teaching careers and a family. They imagined the cozy home they would own in the city, which would of course be walking or biking distance to their jobs in a nearby city school. They talked about starting a family and about extended summer vacations traveling the country with their kids camping, biking, and hiking, like they did themselves as kids. They would even joke about having enough "offspring" to start their own softball team.

Now, some 15 years after their grad school days, the married, 40-year-old Pats have three daughters: Penelope (7), Paige (9), and their oldest, Patrice (11), who they call "Patty." After a few years spent living downtown, they moved with their then-two toddlers and a pregnant Pat to the suburbs into a five-bedroom, newly constructed home with a small yard. To the young family, the home's location was convenient to shopping and chain restaurants and allowed them to get much more house for the money, but it also left them with hefty commutes: more than an hour each way to their jobs at two different high schools across town. So to soften the blow of the long commutes, they splurged and bought a pair of fully loaded mini SUVs.

While they loved being in the classroom, in recent years both Pat and Pat took on roles as administrators at their schools as well. They also decided to start a full-time tutoring business from a room at their neighborhood's local high school during the summer break. The higher administrative salaries and additional income just made sense to them given their current mortgage and car payments, not to mention the family-of-five food bill, cable bill, internet bill, cell phone bills, babysitter bills, and extracurricular fees.

Not surprisingly, the Pats' lives are stressful and far from active or healthy. With three girls, busy full-time jobs, and long daily commutes, this once athletic and energetic couple does not exercise or eat well. As they see it, their schedules simply aren't conducive to either.

On any given weekday for the last several years, the Pats' breakfast consists of a rushed bowl of cereal and toast while getting the three girls up, fed, and out the door in time to make the school bus. They each fill their to-go mug with cream- and sugar-filled coffee and grab a granola bar to get them through their commutes. At work, they like the convenience of the school-provided lunches. Usually on the menu are meatloaf with mashed potatoes and gravy, pizza, tacos, fried chicken nuggets and fries, and always a dessert. And they generally attack the vending machines once or twice a day for a soda and maybe a bag of chips. After work and once the girls have been picked up from the sitter's or their various activities, the norm is to argue as to whose turn it is, as well as what to "make" for dinner, as the meal is never preplanned. More often than not, a drive-through meal, an On-Call Entree delivery, or a frozen lasagna is the solution.

Their postdinner evening is "booked" too, with the girls' homework, their own work approving teachers' lesson plans, and dealing with parent issues, periodic PTA or school board meetings, and developing marketing and tutoring plans for their own business. So a couple of hours of couch time before bed with television or social media (or both simultaneously) is pretty much all their minds can handle (with late-night snacks in hand).

The next day the cycle repeats. The months and years have flown by and the pounds have crept on. Pat and Pat find themselves each 50 pounds or more heavier than they were when they got married. At 5'9", Patrick weighs 222 pounds, and at 5'4" Patricia is 184 pounds. They're not happy with how they look or feel, but neither one makes "changing" a priority.

Unfortunately, the Pats have passed these sedentary habits down to their daughters. The three sweet but shy girls participate in very few truly physical recreational activities or sports. Instead, they spend much of their free time in front of technology. Each of the three girls has their own SmartTablet v10.0, and while Patty had to wait until her tenth birthday to get her own phone, Pat and Pat felt bad for the other two girls, so all three of them have one now.

And since Pat and Pat themselves eat what they desire when they desire it, they put very few food restrictions on their three daughters. They keep their pantry full of sugary cereals, raisin and cinnamon breads, and muffins for their girls' breakfasts; they pack flavored granola bars for their kids' midmorning snacks; they allow them to choose their own school lunches from the cafeteria menu; and they provide them with money for the vending machines in case they get hungry after lunch. The girls also have unlimited access to the pantry and soda supply when everyone gets home from school.

Their oldest, Patty, is at that age where hormones are clearly present and her body is changing. She has become overly self-conscious of her appearance. She knows she doesn't look the same as many of the other girls, particularly the lean, athletic ones. So she says "no" to social situations where she'll be forced to be in less clothing, like pool parties and sleepovers. In the locker room before gym class, she can avoid getting undressed in front of her peers because she hides her gym clothes underneath her school clothes so she can make a "quick change." To make matters worse, she was crushed when she overheard another girl on the bus refer to her as "Fatty Patty." She's since heard those painful words over and over again in her head.

Patty will be 12 in two months. With middle school looming, she's wondering how she's going to fit in with the other girls. Like her parents, she has her own social media accounts and has become obsessed with following the posts of the middle school's most popular kids.

As their daughters have gotten older, Pat and Pat recognize that all three girls carry more weight than their peers and are much heavier than they themselves were as kids. At last summer's wellness visit, the pediatrician scored Patty in the 90th percentile in weight within her age group, and in the 50th percentile in height, and the younger girls had similar scores.

In an effort to combat the girls' weight issues, Pat and Pat signed all three girls up for recreational activities at the start of this past school year: basic dance for little Penelope, beginner gymnastics for Paige, and soccer for Patty, even though she protested. They figured adding some physical activity would do them all some good and would help them shed the extra pounds. Soon into the fall soccer season, however, they noticed that Patty was one of the slowest girls on the field and was having problems keeping up with the other kids in terms of conditioning. Patty often complained of aching knees, but they hoped it was more of an excuse to not play than an actual injury.

But watching their Patty struggle on the field was more than just a concern, it was heartbreaking for Pat and Pat. They thought Patty must be feeling ashamed of how she struggles to keep up, so they decided the best course of action would be private help from a specialized soccer coach.

Patty's private soccer coach turned out to be a bit of a drill sergeant/jerk: he has her running shuttles, suicides, sprints, and more, all with a soccer ball in tow. And as the once-per-week lessons go on for about 6 weeks, the Pats see no visible changes in Patty's performance on the field. Instead, she is complaining even more about her knee pain, becoming more frustrated, and is rapidly losing interest in soccer altogether.

Paige, the middle daughter, is also displaying some physical performance issues in gymnastics class, where she's finding it very difficult to pull herself above the bar or up the bull rope, as she's simply much too heavy.

At Penelope's dance lessons, the seven-year-old finds it hard to get through the entire one-hour class without a break and a snack.

Ironically, after enrolling their girls in physical activities hoping to address their weight gain, Pat and Pat reward their girls after most practices, games, and recitals with a ritual ice cream cone or sundae. And because they're pushed for time, they often resort to a family fast-food dinner when those activities finish up late in the evening.

Dear Patrick and Patricia,

Wake up! You have yet to accept responsibility for Patty, your two other daughters, or yourselves for being overweight. This is not some sort of genetic issue that is attacking your family; they are overweight for the exact same reasons you two are. They eat whatever they want, whenever they want.

You two were not overweight as children, for you were truly recreationally active and spent much of your free time running around the neighborhood with your peers. You were not consumed with technology (since there was not much to be had), and you didn't grow up with massive amounts of processed foods at your fingertips.

You were energetic, fun-loving kids of the 80s, and you were healthy, plain and simple.

But now, Pat and Pat, you are the leaders of your family, and the fact is you have lost control of your own eating habits. Those habits, along with your own sedentary lifestyles, are being passed down to your three lovely little creations. The only way things are going to change for Patty, Paige, and Penelope are for you two to take control of your family's priorities and lead by example.

It will not be easy. Actually, it will kind of suck in the short term, since you're both caught up in the comfort of processed foods, technology, and convenience. But this change will be worth it, and for goodness sake, it's vital for the mental and physical health of your family.

First, sit down with your family (yes, call a family meeting) and discuss the changes that need to take place. Then, seek out the assistance of professional trainers who will help with a well-designed performance training program (rather than a specialized sports coach) along with a nutrition plan based on foods Mother Nature provides. Discuss a shopping list of healthy foods that your family can agree on. Work together on this list to find some compromise, but don't give in too much to the wants of your girls. Remember you two are the leaders, and these girls are used to eating what they want, when they want. That needs to change.

Consider a food-prep day together on the weekend. And how about a small garden, or at minimum vegetable pots and planters? Teach these girls where food comes from (hint: it's not the grocery store), and give them the responsibility and the rewards reaped from this responsibility.

...take control of your family's priorities and lead by example.

And as far as technology goes, Pat and Pat, shame on you for giving your young daughters their own SmartTablets and phones. They're 11, 9, and 7! Pull those devices away from them and spend quality time together away from technology.

Remember your active grad school days when your dreams for family fun included camping, hiking, biking, and summer travel? How have you veered so far off-track? Aren't you missing the physical activity you craved as youngsters and young adults yourselves?

Make changes now. Your oldest daughter, Patty, is fragile, and she is hurting. Recognize this, and help her modify her behaviors and the rest of your family's behaviors, starting at home.

How about Friday night board games and cards over a plate of cut-up veggies and berries? Weekly bike rides and treks? Gardening! Maybe take on a monthly project together like painting a room.

These habits will also save you a tremendous amount of time and money as you won't be forced to cover all the excess technology hardware, software, and monthly charges. Maybe being home a little more and actually being "present" when you are home is just what your daughters need. Ever think those loaded vehicles with the built-in TV screens could be downsized as well? You'd be home a lot more and the stress levels would come way down.

Or you could pull the BS card and teach your children that it's okay to live a comfortable, sedentary life full of gluttonous eating habits and material acquisitions, with the mindset that you should be accepted no matter what size you are. But the world can unfortunately be a mean place, and that also has to be accepted. And again, we're not dealing with genetic issues here, we're dealing with self-inflicted behaviors.

You both must discontinue this gluttonous, sedentary lifestyle and lead by example. Lead those little girls with love, purpose, humility, and faith.

AE

CHAPTER 4

Resolution Randy

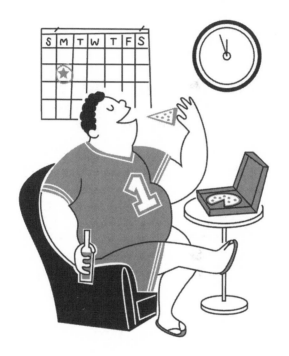

New Year's Day is just around the corner, and Randy is preparing for the first day of his new life. Randy is frustrated with his 34-year-old, 6′1″, 290-pound frame, as well as the stress that comes with his commercial insurance sales job and the high-pressure monthly sales quotas. He's tired physically, and psychologically he's struggling. He reflects frequently on his high school glory days of being a three-sport athlete at 179 pounds as a senior and is determined to get a lean and energetic body back.

This New Year will be the start of the "New Randy" and an end to the red-faced, double-necked, big-bellied, saggy-chested, stiff, sore, and exhausted Randy.

He's already joined Earthy Fitness, where he received the New Year's special of zero money down and $8/month for 12 months. He even upgraded his membership to Earthy Plus, a whopping $14/month, which will give him access to the hundreds of other Earthy Fitness franchises across the country for when he's traveling for work.

With only five days left to the New Year, Randy is pounding down every single one of his favorite fat-, sugar-, and calorie-loaded foods, knowing that a huge sacrifice is coming where he'll make drastic changes to his lifestyle.

When New Year's Eve finally arrives, Randy heads to the grocery store to purchase a large stock of health foods such as low-fat cereals, whole grain breads, low-sodium soups and lunch meats, microwaveable bags of frozen veggies with low-sodium season packets, protein bars, and fruit juices. He also grabs a few succulent goodies such as his favorite cupcakes and frozen pizzas, as he's planning to eat up until midnight and go "cold turkey" from there on.

The next day Randy hits the gym, where he gets acquainted with the machines that work each individual body part, and after a few circuits of each, he grabs 30 minutes on the elliptical machine.

Randy feels great! He's planning to head home now and grab a bowl of low-fat cereal and a bagel with light cream cheese, and begins to plan out the rest of the day and week, up until he gets his first "cheat" day on Sunday. (After his huge sacrifice he feels he'll have earned it.) Randy hits the gym four days that first week, and is eating mostly the items he purchased for his resolution.

But he folds on Thursday evening (Day 3 of the New Year's resolution) when he's out with a group of clients who are of similar age, and the social cocktails turn into an all-night festival that concludes with late-night bar food and more alcohol. Needless to say, Randy has failed his latest resolution as the Day 3 letdown rolls into a weekend of partying.

Randy hasn't thrown the New Year's towel in completely, however, as he thinks to himself that Monday is the perfect time to get back on track. As a matter of fact, Randy promises himself to get on track on most Mondays of the year, as well as the first day of each month. And when the first of the month falls on a Monday, look out! Randy really means it this time. Nonetheless, by the time the end of January rolls around, the hint of a successful New Year's resolution is history.

Thus, Randy now has his sights for transformation set on the upcoming Lenten season, where he'll give up many of the unhealthy foods he likes to consume! His plan of attack is the same. As soon as Lent begins, he will make huge sacrifices in his food intake and begin a consistent regimen of fitness. But in the meantime, he'll load up on all the goodies he can force down, climaxing with an epic "Fat Tuesday" binge for the ages. The following day he's at the gym with the identical approach of a few rounds through the machine circuit, and then off to the elliptical for a good 30-minute sweat. And of course he takes the same approach to his version of sacrificial eating, where he begins the day with low-fat cereal and a piece of whole wheat toast with light butter, a lunch of multi-grain bread and low-sodium lunch meat ham, and dinner is a salad with low-fat dressing, low-fat cheese, and low-sodium croutons along with a can of low-fat chicken noodle soup.

But after 11 days, and that includes a cheat day at Day 5 (hey, Sunday is a cheat day, after all), Randy again loses his focus, this time when he's out with his buddies, which again leads into a weekend of drinking and really poor food selections.

Next up is Easter, so he'll get through the Easter Sunday festivities and "feast" and will commit to getting fit on Monday. Once this resolution dwindles, his new primary target will be following the Memorial Day weekend where he'll consume a massive amount of picnic food and beer, for he knows the next day is the first day of his new life. Then, the week following Independence Day. Next up, postsummer vacation, where the week-long consumption of boardwalk foods and beachside grilling will be his final feasts. After that fails, his next target is Labor Day weekend, where again he'll load up on picnic foods before he enters the days of abstinence. This is followed up with the day after Halloween and then finally right after Thanksgiving. Come full circle, Randy's next target is...what else? The New Year's resolution. But rest assured, Randy will consume an excessive amount of all of his favorites throughout the extended holiday season before that huge commitment begins on January 1st.

Dear Randy,
I realize you have to be hurting emotionally with the more than 100 pounds added to your frame since high school. I'm

sure it weighs on you physically as well. But Randy, your resolution approach to long-term transformation is not rational. You feel as if you are making an insurmountable sacrifice by giving up the gluttonous foods that you eat day in and out, when in reality the foods you choose for your resolution are not doing you any favors. How about the next time you go shopping you try to stock up on fresh veggies rather that the frozen varieties seasoned with oils, sugars, and salt? Fruits such as apples, oranges, and grapes rather than fruit juices. Proteins such as fresh meats and seafood rather than deli lunchmeat, protein bars, and soups. And oats, potatoes, yams, and rice rather than bread, bagels, and cereal.

Randy, in the words of the great Apollo Creed, "There is no tomorrow."

Also, you approach fitness in a half-assed way, where somehow a circuit of strength machines and a hamster wheel is going to give you the lean physique and the physical abilities you crave. Note: you get what you pay for.

Randy, you need to learn what well-programmed performance training is. Even more so, you need to understand the rule of adhering to a nutrition philosophy based on foods that can be fished, grown, and butchered.

And Randy, this whole wait till Monday, or the first of the month, or after the next holiday? Switch it up man— what you're doing isn't working! You are 290 pounds! Shock the world and start on a Friday. Yes, that means you'd eat clean on a Sunday! You haven't even come close to earning a "cheat" day—talk to me in six weeks about a "cheat" day.

Randy, in the words of the great Apollo Creed, "There is no tomorrow."

AE

....

CHAPTER 5

Fitness-Freak Faith

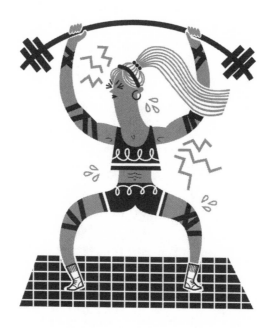

Faith is 36 years old and has been dating 39-year-old Fabian for over seven years. Faith met Fabian eight years ago when he was coaching her first high-intensity group-training class at Warrior Workhouse, which she agreed to try on a whim with a couple of her friends who were members.

Leading up to this chance meeting, Faith had always been active. She competed in gymnastics in elementary and middle school and cheered throughout high school as well as all four years at the Division 3 college she attended. Faith continued her active lifestyle at a local fitness franchise after beginning her career in the HR field, where she ran three times each week on the treadmill, took a couple of body-sculpting classes each week, and almost always tried any of the new class offerings her fitness center introduced.

But this class with Fabian was different! Faith was hooked midway through her first workout, with sweat pouring off of her entire body as he barked out commands of pull-ups on the gymnastic rings, squat jumps to maximum height, medicine-ball throws, sprints, and more. Faith's gymnastics and cheer background came in super handy, as she was crushing her friends as well as many of the regulars in this timed event. Her body felt like jelly after the workout, and she awoke the next day to an unbelievable amount of soreness, but her sense of accomplishment and endorphins were through the roof. The following day she was back at class ready to compete and also ready to show off a bit for the super ripped and fit Fabian.

It didn't take long for Fabian to notice the attractive, high-energy, and athletic new student in his 5:30 p.m. class. And it took him even less time to make his move. Within a few weeks, Faith and Fabian were on their first date. It turned out that Fabian had joined the same warehouse gym three years prior to Faith when he was looking to get back into shape after working in the sedentary and entertainment-filled mortgage industry since graduating college. Fabian got hooked on this high-intensity training as well, for he was quite the athlete in high school and picked up on this "athletic" stuff pretty easily. It wasn't long before Fabian started entering different fitness competitions as well as becoming a coach who taught fitness classes. He loved that as a bonus, teaching got him a free membership to the gym.

As Faith's relationship with Fabian started to get a little more real, so did her desire to train competitively, and it wasn't long before she herself entered her first fitness competition. Faith placed 18th in that first competition, and from then on she was an absolute animal in the gym, training six and sometimes seven days per week, with muscles on top of her muscles to prove it.

Faith was on top of the world because her training left her feeling great about herself, and her relationship with Fabian was perfect. They shared all the same interests in training and eating, and they just so happened to love their own and each other's ripped, muscular physiques. Their lives revolved around their training and eating, and most of the friends and couples they hung out with were cut from the same fabric. The more competitions Faith entered, the higher she finished, which sparked a flame deep inside to want to be The Best. So she trained even harder, sometimes twice a day.

But just as Faith had muscles upon muscles as a result of her training, she also had injury upon injury as a direct result of her training. Two years after the start of her competitive training days, Faith developed tendinitis in both elbows that likely stemmed from pull-up after pull-up, which she was able to endure with a corticosteroid pack and dual training sleeves. In the next couple of years, things got a little worse when she had minor surgery to repair a tear in her shoulder that likely arose from high-volume overhead lifts. In addition, she got to wear "the token boot" multiple times to deal with the stress fractures in her feet that likely manifested from excessive amounts of jumps and runs.

In the ensuing years, things got much worse as Faith had to cope with a couple of bulging discs in her back that the doctors felt were a direct result of the excessive loads on her frame, which essentially limited her ability to perform most of the activities she fell in love with. Unfortunately for Faith, there wasn't a band or brace that could mask the radiating nerve pain running down her legs.

Now only in her mid-30s, Faith has been fighting the realization that not only have her event competition days come to an end, so has her aggressive style of training within the classes themselves. As for her man Fabian, he, too, has been plagued by injuries and trains very little on his own. He has resorted to mostly coaching verbally, as his late-30s body is simply unable to instruct many of the complex movements that came so easily to him in his 20s.

Ironically, Faith and Fabian have switched their memberships to the same fitness franchise that Faith was a member of eight years ago. The same fitness franchise they ridiculed for being inferior to their elite way of training when they were in the prime of their competitive years. But now their cardio is limited to the upright bikes and elliptical machines as their injuries related to their excessive running and jumping do not allow for much treadmill work. And while they still are able to perform a few fancy feats in the free-weight room compared to the average member, they are a far cry from max efforts under the squat bar and the pull-up area, and the fast moving Olympic lifts are but a distant memory.

Furthermore, Faith is actually dealing with some emotional issues with her own personal image and physical fitness, as she is no longer able to maintain muscle volume due to her inability to train excessively, and she feels Father Time is closing in. Now at age 36, after years of focusing on herself, she's just now starting to think about marriage and a baby and is concerned she waited too long. Fabian is dealing with some personal vanity issues himself and is wondering if he's too old to be a first-time dad.

Dear Faith and Fabian,

You have been struck with the addiction of exercise that so many have before you. Just like a professional athlete, the ability to perform at a high level comes to an end in the late 20s and early 30s, with a few exceptions. We so often see our favorite all-stars experience their first hamstring pull, then another and another as they enter their final years of competition. Sometimes it's even more unfortunate, like a career-ending Achilles tear that's hard to watch on the replay, yet is shown over and over. Faith, you and Fabian were dominant in your 20s because you were...well, you were in your 20s. But just like real athletes who competed in real sports for years on end, you now have the wear and tear on your body to deal with from the excessive and intense workouts you've taken part in for years on end.

But the ho-hum health-club approach is not your answer. You need to seek out a system of training that can heal much of your damage and allow you to progress forward in a safe and sustainable way. Neither of you are spring chickens, and while your age is certainly not a death sentence, you need to train smart going forward and leave the day in, *day out, competitive-style of training to the young and re-silient (although those young and resilient will need to pay the piper one day as well if they take the same approach you two did).*

And by all means, if you have personal fitness goals and objectives that you want to meet, go after them. If you want to match that highest jump or that best lift of your past, please have at it. But choose your goals wisely— one at a time and within rea-son!—and embrace the aging

...embrace the aging process by training strategically, safely, and sustainably.

process by training strategically, safely, and sustainably. While training within this type of system may not result in you being the best in the gym or the fittest in your county, this approach will allow you to be powerful, strong, and mobile, and your cardio will be well developed, now and for years to come.

Faith and Fabian, if you want to continue a life togeth-er as a team, make a real commitment to each other and get married. Build a family and learn from your mistakes by teaching your children the lifelong lessons of training sustainably.

AE

CHAPTER 6

Supplement Sam

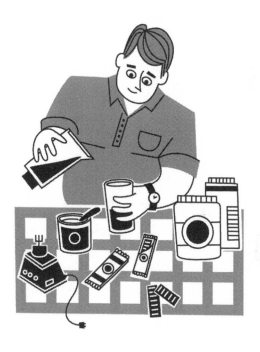

am is a classic corporate musclehead, and looking at a typical day for him reveals just that. While his business-suited body sits trapped in his cubicle from 9:00 to 5:00, his mind, as well as his heart, longs for the gym. From the minute he wakes up until he goes to bed, Sam is thinking about his workouts, his body, and his beloved supplements. He obsesses about how his magic pills, powders, and products will help him add more muscle and look more ripped for the potential ladies in his life—particularly Samantha.

Sam wakes up most mornings and mixes his specially engineered protein powder (his rationale: super muscle-building properties) with kefir (his rationale: huge in probiotics), exotic fruit (his rationale: high in rare antioxidants), and special nuts (his rationale: increased testosterone) from a faraway country. He then pops a couple pieces of what has to be organic sprouted bread into the toaster and spreads it with a couple tablespoons of natural peanut butter. Before leaving for work, he prepares his hyper-caffeinated coffee blend (his rationale: huge energy) with a couple teaspoons of natural sugar cane (his rationale: more energy) along with medium-chain triglyceride (MCT) oil (his rationale: huge fat-burning properties). Shortly after he gets to work, Sam downs his first protein-rich energy bar (his rationale: more muscle-building properties) and maybe another cup of coffee, along with another dose of the natural cane sugar and MCT oil and his daily dose vitamin pack. When it's time for lunch, Sam hits the local sushi hotspot, since it offers an array of muscle-building protein sources, and orders the two-tuna, lightly battered and fried tempura roll special.

By midafternoon, Sam realizes he needs another protein-rich bar (his rationale: more muscle-building properties) as well as the 16 oz. sugar-added, caffeine-loaded, prepackaged energy drink he has each day at this time for an afternoon jolt. Sam feels great and is firing on all cylinders. He takes a minute to look around the cubicle jungle and wonders how his fellow coworkers (he thinks: the poor saps) can get through the day with only their brown bag lunches and afternoon coffee break.

As a matter of fact, around the office, Sam is often

referred to as Super Stud Sam, as he looks huge in his business suits and many of his admiring fellow employees view him as their at-work fitness expert. And Sam, being Sam, eats this attention up, gladly sharing his tips for muscle success at every opportunity.

Now it's five o'clock, and that means quitting time, which means he'll be at the gym in another 30 minutes, so he needs to fuel up on an amino-acid-rich preworkout protein shake (his rationale: even more muscle-building protein) to make sure he's primed for his workouts.

Sam hits the gym and is eager to meet up with his training partners, Seth and Samantha. Sam and Samantha have had a thing for each other for several months, but both have similar insecurities and can't seem to pull the trigger to act on their interests. The three amigos catch up on the latest gym gossip while working multiple sets of chest exercises along with super sets of biceps and triceps.

After the workout, Sam and his crew hit the smoothie bar at the gym for a bit to down another postworkout, protein-rich recovery shake (his rationale: to ensure they don't compromise any valuable muscle from the intense chest and arm workout they just completed) and to get a few laughs as they watch all the amateurs and two- or three-timers a week in the gym go at it.

Soon it's dinner time, and Sam knows he's been "on" all day with his program, so he'll make sure he has a calorie-rich, manly meal to ensure he continues to grow his muscles. That often entails a ten-ounce steak with sauce, a baked potato with butter and sour cream, and some veggies with a little more butter, along with a couple beers (his rationale: it's manly), and onward he goes on his journey.

Before bed Sam makes sure he has a protein-rich shake that is specifically touted for late evening, providing slow-releasing protein as he sleeps (his rationale: once again, to help preserve and build precious muscle).

Ironically however, with all this focus on Sam and his body, Sam never really seems to change much in his appearance. Without a doubt, Sam is a beefier guy than the normal Joe. After all, he hits the gym five days each week after work to pump iron. But something's just not jiving; while Sam has some decently sized arms and a barrel chest, he seems to lack any real definition, his face is puffy, and he also has a pretty big belly.

Sam himself is well aware of this, for every night when he goes to shower he catches a glimpse of himself in the mirror. He looks pumped in the tight t-shirt he still has on from the gym and for a brief moment, is content with his day. But then Sam strips down for the shower and catches another glimpse of his 5′10″, 225-pound, 25-percent-body-fat self (by the way, this equates to 56 pounds of fat) and is deflated. He thinks to himself: how is it possible that he has this huge belly, these love handles, this excess fat on his chest, and fat in his legs? He's convinced he's doing everything right. He knows all the super-secret tricks: he trains right, eats right, and takes all the special protein shakes, protein bars, and vitamins. He's also upset that his shoulders and elbows are in chronic pain, and he's even more upset that this pain is restricting his ability in the gym to push as much weight as he used to.

Once Sam's out of the shower, he pops open his laptop and starts researching for a fat-burning supplement and joint formula to compliment everything else he does right.

There's got to be an answer—a pill, product, or powder—available online.

Dear Sam,

You're stuck somewhere out in the "in-between land." You want to change, and so you're willing to throw money at the latest, cutting-edge product, and of course, you're willing to pump iron. But you're not committed to making the true sacrifices necessary to obtain that lean, muscular version of the Sam you desire.

Sam, it's time for a reality check.

You are essentially "all show and no go." You talk the talk but you don't walk the walk. You're constantly cutting corners and taking shortcuts rather than making the real lifestyle changes necessary to get that lean, muscular physique you envision.

First, you need to strongly consider cutting out many of these formulated protein shakes and protein bars, and take a more disciplined, humble approach to food by consuming real foods prepared in a plain and what is often perceived as boring fashion. Try a couple of poached eggs (an excellent and natural protein source) and a bowl of boiled oats with blueberries in the morning, a piece of fruit with nuts for snacks, a piece of steamed fish or

> You're constantly cutting corners and taking shortcuts rather than making real lifestyle changes.

grilled chicken (again natural protein sources) along with a bowl of steamed rice or a baked yam, and a large bowl of steamed veggies for both lunch and dinner. If you really need that slow-releasing protein overnight, you can add in a bowl of plain cottage cheese in the late evening. And sure, if you feel like you need a protein shake postworkout, this option could be justified here.

But now, man, let's address your workout routines. Sam, you need to step out of the 80s. Training chest and arms day in and day out will do little to give you the look you want (but a lot of what you don't want like elbows full of arthritis). Have you ever heard of legs? Core? Posterior chain? Cardio? Recovery? Sam you need a comprehensive training program where you'll focus on strength, power, mobility, and energy system development.

Sam, you can't keep on rationalizing with your current "manly" workouts and your supplement-filled approach. If you want those big yet undefined arms and barreled yet saggy pecs to ever transform, you'll need to get out of your own way and be willing to know what you don't know. And who knows, maybe Samantha will join you in your journey...wink, wink!

And one last thing, Sam. You're simply not that big of a dude. You graduated high school at 178 pounds. You haven't added 47 pounds of muscle over the years—most of it is fat. Drop 30 of that added fat weight and you'll be down to 195 pounds—accept this and look more like an athlete rather than Johnny Bravo.

AE

CHAPTER 7

Travel-Ball Tammy

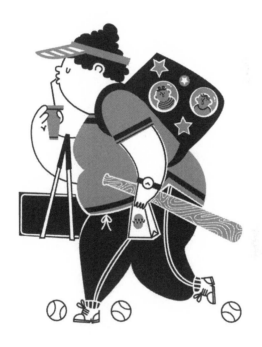

Tammy is in her late 30s and is absolutely all about her son, Timmy. Timmy is a 10-year-old "phenom" baseball player who competes year-round on various indoor and outdoor "Elite" travel teams. Tammy and her husband Tommy spare no expense when it comes to their little prodigy, paying for private hitting and catching lessons throughout the year.

Tammy's life essentially revolves around Timmy's baseball tournament schedule and private lessons. In her mind, his success equates to her success, and she thrives on it. "Classic Tammy," as those who know her would say, is a mom who can be found pacing behind the practice cage, with a heavily caffeinated whipped latte in hand, barking out commands to her son to perform the way his private coaches are instructing.

Tammy and her husband Tommy travel almost every weekend of the summer season to elite tournaments to watch Timmy and his team compete in local, regional, and even national tournaments. Tammy and Tommy also have a younger son, Tommy Jr., who is on the newly formed tee-ball travel circuit as well, and it looks as though he may be the next natural ball player in the family.

At ten, Timmy shows a good bit of athleticism for his age and is one of the larger kids on the team, both in height, but also in weight (and it should be noted this "weight" is not just muscle). It's clear he's one of the better players on his team, hitting a couple of home runs each year and making a few nice throws to second from his catcher's position. Tammy and Tommy couldn't be prouder of their boy and have visions of Division 1 schools knocking on their doors in a few years.

Tammy is the Team Mom of Timmy's travel team, where she organizes and delegates the food and beverage lists for "tailgating/refueling" in between games, designating which of the other players' parents will bring the pulled pork, the buns, the chips, the hot dogs, the burgers, the brownies, the cookies, and the soda. The young athletes are sometimes playing three or four games in a day, and their parents believe it's important they refuel when they have downtime in between play.

Fast-forward three years to Timmy, now age 13. Many of the other boys Timmy once towered over have hit puberty, so Timmy is no longer one of the tallest boys on his team. But he is still the heaviest—and the slowest.

To make matters worse, Timmy really doesn't love baseball anymore.

He dreads the grind that his parents have set up for him and actually is beginning to resent them. Furthermore, he's coming into an age where his hormones are all over the place. He's becoming aware of his self-image, comparing himself to other boys and taking an interest in girls. It should also be noted that little Tommy Jr. is currently the prodigy, as he is now 10 years old and following in the footsteps of his older brother both in height and in weight.

Team Mom Tammy is 42 years old, is 5'5" tall, and weighs 208 pounds. Her husband Tommy, who is also 42 years old, is 5'8" tall and weighs 235 pounds. Tammy and Tommy never thought to consider the fact that genetics was going to play a role in Timmy's growth—he would most likely never be a tall fellow—or that their family's eating habits would play a factor in Timmy's girth. Nor did they consider how the pattern of eating "what he wants, when he wants," just as his parents do, has become his habit at an awkward age of 13—and sadly, the same will be true for little Tommy Jr.

Regarding her own self-image, Tammy is embarrassed by the way she looks, but she is so busy with Timmy and Tommy Jr.'s schedules that taking care of herself seems frivolous. Tommy is not much happier as he knows he's put on weight, and though he's married, he feels lonely. To make matters worse, they don't find each other physically attractive any longer. With tournaments and associated hotel stays almost every weekend, they are eating at fast food restaurants frequently and tailgating at games. Timmy and Tommy's practice schedules during the week have them running as well, so the fast food habits are the rule rather than the exception at this point.

Tammy and Tommy's version of intimacy is sitting down together with calendars in hand over a take-out meal of fried food, navigating the boys' travel schedules, lessons, practices, and homework. As far as they are concerned, their life is their kids, and connecting with one another on a romantic level is a thing of the past.

Essentially, Tammy and Tommy are no longer a couple. Instead, they have transitioned into a business relationship where they serve as dual sports agents for their boys.

Dear Tammy and Tommy,

In your quest to live your dreams through your children, you are oblivious to the fact that you are leading your boys down a path of detrimental behaviors that they will likely spend the rest of their lives trying to reverse—and worse, they may even resent you for it all.

The unhealthy food and drink that you are supplying to "fuel" your young athletes on game days is actually just serving to quench your own desires. Hot dogs, cookies, brownies, and chips for "refuel" purposes? Seriously?

You are the parents, and you are responsible for their food choices. Did you ever consider something as simple as a piece of fruit and a handful of nuts between games? Or a chilled smoothie of plain yogurt, frozen berries, coconut water, and a teaspoon of honey? Or something more robust for extended breaks, such as a sealable bowl of diced, grilled chicken breast and steamed rice pilaf with avocado? These eating habits sure as heck would be more in line with those of most professional athletes! And as for the frequent out-of-town travel and hotels, not to mention the reliance on fast food, you're again sabotaging your children due to your own desires and wants for convenience.

As far as Timmy's skill development, you invested significant resources with private lessons for hitting and catching, but little to no development on his speed and performance training, his nutrition, or his rest and recovery. All of these elements are required to foster a top-notch athlete, even at the youngest levels.

...you need to find balance... and let your boys be boys.

And guys, honestly: if it happens that Timmy or Tommy Jr. are truly prodigies, it will become clearly apparent without the grinding travel schedule that you started when they were 6 years old. While hard work undoubtedly plays a role in development and the success of an athlete, genetics cannot be overlooked in the making of a prodigy. Ask yourselves, as neither of you is over 5' 8", do you expect either of your sons to reach a height that Division 1 schools are looking for?

In addition to being the focus of your time outside of work, your boys' travel-ball tournaments are your primary source for social events and family bonding. At this point, Timmy doesn't even enjoy the game. Are you so invested *that his feelings don't enter into your scholarship equation?*

Tammy and Tommy, you need to find balance. You need to let your boys be boys, where they climb trees, shoot hoops, play a few different sports, and spend time simply being active together as a family. Perhaps you can take weekly hikes and bike rides together.

You also need to find time for one another, taking care of yourselves and each other, for each other as well as for your boys.

AE

CHAPTER 8

Gluten-Free Glen

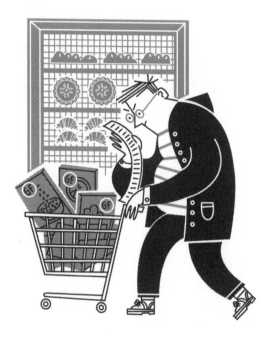

Glen is in his late 50s and has struggled with his weight for as long as he can remember. He has tried numerous diets and fads over his lifetime, with varying degrees of short-term success. He's even taken his wife and his three children along for some of his dieting adventures, hoping that by getting the whole family involved in his struggle, he would be bound to reach his goal. Glen's latest approach, and one that he's convinced will be the ultimate answer, is a gluten-free diet.

Glen has been doing his *own* research and now believes the reason he's been overweight for so long is his intolerance to gluten, which is a protein found in wheat, rye, and barley. He's been reading the gluten-free social media posts and forums of others' stories and their battles with weight and is starting to see the similarities he shares.

He has suddenly realized that gluten has been the culprit and that his numerous approaches to weight loss (low-carbohydrate, low-fat, high-protein, fasting, detoxing, and so on) were a waste of time. Glen believes that it's his sensitivity to gluten that has caused him to be 50+ pounds overweight and has been the undermining factor all along when he battled his weight with those other approaches.

Convinced he has the answer, he asks his doctor to test him for gluten sensitivity. Oddly enough, Glen is actually somewhat disappointed by his doctor's news that his gluten sensitivity is mild at best. Regardless, Glen dives headfirst into his new gluten-free lifestyle, and convinces his wife and kids to do the same.

Glen and his family cut out the frequent staples of their household, items such as bagels, waffles, muffins, rolls, cereals, creamy dressings, frozen spaghetti alfredo meals, and so on. He consumes mostly lean proteins, steamed vegetables, and boiled starches like rice and potatoes. And in turn he finds himself dropping weight and feeling full of energy and focus within the first week.

However, within two weeks, Glen takes a familiar approach to past diet attempts by preparing a shopping list of items that he enjoys, just gluten-free versions of them. He purchases gluten-free cookies, gluten-free brownies, gluten-free waffles, gluten-free breads, gluten-free pizza, gluten-free spaghetti, and gluten-free beer. He even found the gluten-free version of his favorite weekend treat, mac and cheese!

But after about six weeks of his gluten-free campaign, just as he has with other diets, Glen has actually put on *more* weight, and this time it's another eight pounds. In addition, his monthly grocery bill has almost doubled with this diet!

Dear Glen,

If you're trying to lose weight and want to have a lean physique, why are you consuming so many processed foods? I know the answer, Glen—and deep down, so do you. Just like so many others, you have sabotaged your approach to healthy eating with rationalizations: "These cookies are gluten-free, they must be okay for my diet." Or, "I can eat as much mac and cheese as I want as long as it's the gluten-free kind." But Glen, these gluten-free processed choices, like their counterparts, are full of excess sugars and various flours. And to boot, they come with a mighty price tag!

Just as you did with your other fads, you have figured out a way to push the limits on this "foolproof meal plan" to the point where it is deemed ineffective.

Yes, Glen, gluten resistance for some folks is very real! A small percentage of the population have a serious autoimmune condition called celiac disease where the consumption of gluten can cause significant damage to the small intestine. Those living with celiac disease have to be very careful not to consume products with gluten, such as wheat, rye, and barley. They face quite a daunting task since it's not just foods like breads, cereals, sauces, soups, beer, and whiskey, but also products such as certain medications and even toothpastes. Furthermore, some of those with celiac disease have to be careful with cross-contamination, avoiding foods that were processed in a plant that also processes wheat, rye, or barley products, and even have to avoid using a toaster that toasts products with gluten.

But Glen, your doctor confirmed that you did not have celiac, but rather a mild level of gluten sensitivity, just as a good percentage of the population does, with minor issues such as bloating, gas, and other ailments.

Stop blaming the gluten, Glen.

So is gluten the real culprit in your weight gain?

No, Glen. You are overweight because of the high-fat, chemical-laden and/or high-sugar products you love to eat: brownies, pastries, pizzas, wings, and fast foods. Whether or not they happen to have gluten in them is inconsequential.

However, if you're going to take a run with the gluten-free approach, you can still be quite successful. First you need to back away from the gluten-free cookies and other processed goodies. Then you should consider grains such as quinoa and various rice blends, potatoes, yams, oats, lean proteins such as fish and turkey, fats such as olive oil and nuts, and all fruits and vegetables—all of these are a "go." Consuming gluten-free foods like these, prepared in a plain and simple fashion, will surely help you drop that weight you so desperately desire to lose (just like it did for you in Week 1, Glen!)

Glen, you will start to conquer your long-standing battle with your weight when you decide to accept that the answer to a lean body is as simple as predominantly eating foods that can be fished, grown, or butchered, in an unadulterated state, combined with proper performance training, over an extended period of time.

Stop blaming the gluten, Glen.

AE

CHAPTER 9

Artificial Anna

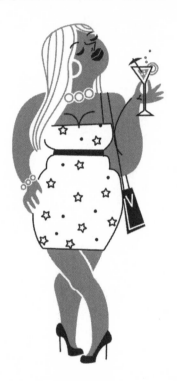

Anna is a 49-year-old mother of two grown children who is now married to her third husband, Andrew, a very high-powered bank executive. Andrew is 14 years older and is set to retire next year as the president of the largest bank in the city. Anna's two children were had with her first husband, Antonio, whom she met in Europe when she was taking modeling classes. Antonio was the son of an Italian sports-car tycoon. Anna's marriage with Antonio ended when the children were young, with a large estate built for the kids, but Anna herself did not fare so well due to a prenup.

Anna's second marriage was to Arthur, the owner of a national contracting company, whom she married in her early 30s. Anna lived a life of high rolling with Arthur, but that marriage ended when Anna was in her early 40s, and again Anna did not fare well due to another prenup.

Anna then met Andrew, a widower, whose first wife passed away in her mid-50s. She married him shortly thereafter—this time with no prenup.

Anna has been obsessed with her appearance as far back as she can remember. She was her high school's homecoming queen, modeled throughout her college years, and even landed a few somewhat lucrative modeling gigs during her stint in Europe. As a matter of fact, she met her first husband Antonio when she was hired to model for his father's line of sports cars.

The birth of her children took a slight toll on her body, but she was young, and her body bounced back rather easily for her (with the help of some minor cosmetic work after each child). In no time Anna was able to gain back her model-like figure, but as she aged and her desire for the finer things in life increased, particularly the finer foods, Anna's body did not rebound as quickly as it did in her youth. By the time she was in her early 30s, Anna felt that a breast augmentation would boost her self-confidence and distract from the pounds she had gained.

With her second marriage, Anna had her breasts done again after a chance encounter with Arthur's first wife, Annabel, when she discovered Annabel's breasts were larger than hers. With money to burn and approaching 40,

Anna began to have some work done on her face as she felt she was beginning to look weathered. After she married Andrew, minor liposuction and facial work procedures became the norm.

At a quick glance, when Anna is out on the town and dressed to kill, she appears to be a bit of a blonde bombshell. With blonde hair, full, injected lips, and a curvy body (particularly upstairs), Anna appears to be quite striking. But there's a hidden secret that Anna knows all too well. When she undresses, she struggles with what she sees. There are scars from her breast augmentation and her liposuction, and she seems to have added fat in areas all around where fat had been removed. Her ankles, calves, and thighs are full of dimples from inches of fat; her arm fat seems to flap in the wind; her hips and stomach appear to be full of cellulite; her face is bloated around her thinned nose and puffed-up lips; and she can't bear to look at her bare self. While Anna still yearns to be desired by a man, she takes comfort in knowing Andrew has never been driven much in a sexual manner, but rather simply enjoys her "company."

Possibly the most concerning, Anna is beginning to wonder if she's a functioning alcoholic, because she finds herself having a glass or two of wine with some dark chocolate every afternoon, and each night when she and Andrew dine out, Anna generally averages two martinis and shares a bottle of wine with Andrew.

So with all of these body image issues, Anna is planning her go-to strategy: more plastic surgery—this time on her face with a brow lift in hopes of getting her youthful appearance back.

As far as Anna's nutrition goes, she half-heartedly

attempts to eat healthily. She starts the day with a smoothie of avocado, organic soy protein powder, Acai berry juice, and a whole grain bagel with natural peanut butter. She snacks on a dark chocolate-flavored protein bar after her midmorning workouts, and then generally heads to the spa, where she'll vary from day to day with either a massage, hair coloring, pedicures, manicures, or tanning. (*Because if you can't tone it, tan it.*)

After the spa appointments, she only has time for a quick lunch where she and her imported sports car hit up the fast food drive-through for a burger and fries.

Back home, she relaxes with her wine and dark chocolate as she waits for Andrew to come home so they can decide together where they'll go for dinner.

A typical dinner out for Anna and Andrew may be lobster with butter sauce, filet mignon with béarnaise sauce, buttered and breaded Dover sole, and sides such as lobster mac and cheese, bacon-encrusted Brussels sprouts, and mashed red potatoes with heavy cream. They rarely pass on desserts such as tiramisu cheesecake, French macaroons, crème brûlée, or Anna's personal favorite, chocolate volcano cake. And weekend breakfasts are at the club with Andrew, where she'll often have quiche Lorraine with local, farm-fresh sausage links.

Anna spares no expense when it comes to exercise. She has hired the most sought-after "mobile trainer" in the area who shows up five times a week for an at-home "workout." These workouts are mostly a chat session, where Anna dishes gossip on many of the other wives from the old money neighborhood. In addition, Anna doesn't like to sweat, so the workouts are kept at a very low throttle with some basic stretching, a little bit of dumbbell work, and a 15-minute walk on the treadmill, where again she dishes more of what's wrong with the world. Two days per week they simply walk in the local park, where—again—it's largely a chat session.

Anna loves having the ability Andrew affords her, and Andrew is happy to have such a striking woman at his side, as he loves the feeling of power. She enjoys her home in the old money suburbs, and she loves her country club lifestyle and her ability to do what she wants when she wants. But in reality, Anna is very unhealthy and unhappy—and counting on the next round of surgery to fix it all.

Dear Anna,

It's sad to see the vain and shallow life you lead. The great genetics you inherited have gone awry not just with age, but with a spoiled approach to food. Rather than respect your body and the aging process, you have continued with the "buy a body" cosmetic approach. Anna, no matter how wealthy you are, you cannot defy Mother Nature.

Anna, you live a life of luxury as your body decays around you.

But it's not too late, Anna. The cosmetic work is done, so let's just accept that. But if you want to obtain a lean resemblance of what you once were, you are going to have to change your materialistic ways and forfeit your "Anna gets what Anna wants" lifestyle. You'll need to eat foods that can be fished, grown, and butchered, prepared in a plain and simple manner. And it might be time to fire that high-priced $150/hour trainer who's willing to allow you to dictate the pace, and instead commit to following a well-designed training program with much more conviction and effort. Also, you should consider seeing a counselor about your drinking habits to ensure you don't have a bigger problem.

Anna, you have continued to live a constant life of luxury as your body decays around you. Come down off that privileged pony you're riding and approach life more humbly. Stop allowing your world to revolve around artificial means of beautification, and accept that no matter how wealthy we are, we're all simply human.

And lastly, Anna, while some may have fancier pants, we all still put our pants on one leg at a time.

AE

CHAPTER 10

Marathon Marvin

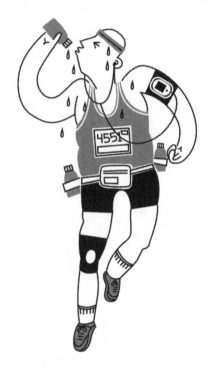

Marvin is about to turn 46. He's married to Mary, is the father of three girls, and works in management for an area mechanical contractor. He's in quite the funk presently, as he's 45 pounds heavier than he was when he graduated high school, and he's recovering from an infection following a knee replacement that became necessary due to exercise, of all things.

Marvin's running career began in his mid-30s when he joined a local fitness center chain to help lose some fat and to get back into shape after he found himself with an unwanted 30 pounds and was given the official title of "dad bod" by his oldest daughter.

When he initially joined the gym, he followed the traditional fitness center script, clipboard in hand, moving from strength machine to strength machine, logging reps and sets, then finishing up with 10 minutes of walking on the treadmill.

After a couple of weeks, Marvin was feeling a little better about himself, but most of it was coming from the additional time he was spending on the treadmill. Marvin ran track in high school, so with each workout, he would instinctively up the time and speed controls on the "tread," which eventually turned into a light running pace.

Not long after that, Marvin found himself skipping the strength machine circuit altogether and eventually working up to three miles on the treadmill three-to-four times each week. Between the running and drastically reduced calorie intake—eating mostly just fruits, salads and other vegetables—the weight was pouring off of Marvin, and he was feeling great!

Marvin went as far as to do some research online to help him design a running program that would get him prepared for a local 10k event. He followed this program to perfection, upping his running to a solid five days per week. And come race day, Marvin finished in the 40th percentile of his age group and felt as if he could walk on water!

After the sense of accomplishment of completing his first 10k, Marvin joined a running group where they met up six mornings per week to run anywhere from five to ten miles each session, and the group started running together in 10k races and even half marathons.

Marvin was amazed that within less than a year, he managed to lose 35 pounds and felt a sense of endorphin release every time he finished a run. He then set his sights on his first marathon.

His training reached an all-time high in volume as he prepared for his marathon, though he experienced a few setbacks along the way, with a minor hip injury and some plantar fascia issues in his feet. But Marvin was tough— "a runner"—always thinking back to his high school days of grinding it out, and managed to get past the injuries and complete his first marathon (of many to come) before his 40th birthday.

Over the next few years, Marvin went after his bucket lists of running events across the eastern seaboard, and he filled his office with his registration bib numbers and race day tee-shirt giveaways hanging on his wall. Marvin was at an all-time high emotionally and an all-time low in weight. He almost looked sickly, as he had lost 40 pounds.

By his early 40s, Marvin began to experience more significant injuries related to his running. He's had to wear a boot for a stress fracture in his foot, had a couple of scopes of his right knee, and underwent a more serious surgery to repair a torn ligament. Marvin's orthopedic surgeon urged him to discontinue his running, but Marvin thought to himself, "I'm an athlete" and continued to rehab those surgeries and injuries the only way he knew how, and that was to begin running again. Unfortunately, on his 45th birthday, as he was attempting to complete the nation's most premier marathon, Marvin heard a large pop and felt a huge pain shoot up his leg.

Turns out the knee could no longer be scoped, and Marvin's running career would come to a forceful end when it became clear a knee replacement was imminent.

Tonight, on the eve of his 46th birthday and a year after his fateful last marathon, Marvin is staring his "new normal" right in the face. He's gained all the weight back that he lost, and more! And he just dealt with a risky infection following his knee replacement surgery that he's lucky to have hurdled. He never thought it could happen to him, but now Marvin is fighting with the realization that his running career has crossed its last finish line, just like it had for so many of his 10K buddies.

Dear Marvin,

Here's the thing (and hearing this may hurt more than your latest knee surgery): during your running career you really were never all that healthy. Sure, your cardiovascular system was fit, as you were really good at running eight-to-nine-minute miles, mile after mile. But your lower extremities were taking an absolute beating, and you were running yourself into a world of dysfunction. In addition, you essentially lost a large amount of muscle tissue as you trained excessively with your running program, performed no resistance exercise, and didn't come close to eating enough calories to support your running addiction.

So you are in a bad place right now, just as countless other runners have had to come to this realization for one overuse reason or another. But there's good news if you're willing to venture outside of your running mentality. (Well, at this point you have no choice.) Your situation can be reversed. And if you listen, you could actually reach a level of true performance that you have yet to experience. You'll have to accept that your long-distance running career is over, but a world of strength, power, mobility, and various energy systems' development awaits you, as well as a whole new approach to food, where you'll consume "bountiful" amounts of food that Mother Nature provides in a plain and simple fashion.

...during your running career you really were never all that healthy.

Tomorrow you turn 46. Make your birthday the start of a new "race." With a consistent, confident approach to strategic, safe, and sustainable training, you'll be a new, high-performing, lean, healthy man by your next birthday!

AE

CHAPTER 11

Traditions Teresa

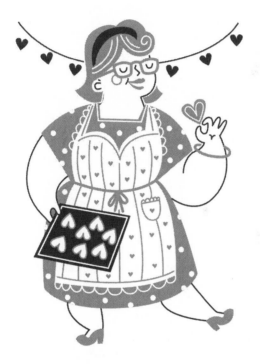

Teresa is in her mid-50s and has multiple health issues, is significantly overweight (officially considered "obese" on the BMI chart), and deals with numerous orthopedic problems, including a knee replacement, a hip replacement, chronic foot pain, and an ankle problem. Teresa is also on both blood pressure and cholesterol medication.

Teresa is one of the sweetest and most trusting ladies you will ever meet and is close to retiring after 30 years as an elementary school librarian and arts and crafts teacher. It's as if she could step right out of a television series featuring 1950s Americana.

Teresa married her college boyfriend very early in her twenties, but the marriage lasted only for a year after she discovered that her then-husband, Tony, had been having a fling with Teresa's roommate in college—and unfortunately, their affair heated up again just a few months after Teresa's and Tony's wedding. Teresa was crushed and has never remarried. Since she never had any children of her own, she has been like a second mother to many of her students throughout the years. Teresa is a natural when it comes to arts and crafts, and her students absolutely adore her.

But Teresa is best known by her students for her sweet treats: the freshly baked cookies every Friday, her hot cocoa during the cold winter months, her sweetened iced tea during the warm spring months, her Christmas cutout sugar cookies during the holiday season, her jelly bean-filled basket at Easter, her Valentine chocolates, and her back-to-school fall pumpkin rolls.

Teresa comes from a large family who loves to cook. Her parents and her grandparents adhered to the tradition of big family meals with rich, hearty homemade ingredients. For *extra* special occasions like holidays, birthdays, confirmations, communions, baptisms, graduations, showers, picnics—and even more recently celebrated, "gender reveal parties" (yeah, that's a thing now)—Teresa makes a trip to the trendy boutique bakery for their signature breads, rolls, tortes, cookies, and cupcakes as a supplement to her own baked creations. And when she needs to step up her "side dish" options for larger family functions, she hits up her favorite authentic Italian deli for their catered stuffed shells, rigatoni, and wedding soup.

The food-centric traditions started early in Teresa's life, as did her weight gain. But these traditions became a part of Teresa's identity (as did her weight), and the thought of having an event without "tradition" was inconceivable to her.

Not surprisingly, Teresa is unhappy with her weight, and for that matter, the state of her overall health. To counter her weight, she has joined four or five gyms over the years, each time burning up the treadmills, elliptical riders, and stationary bikes for hours on end. Teresa has also trekked the local, environmentally protected trails with friends periodically, where the terrains vary, and the feelings of accomplishment are high. Over the years, Teresa has also joined many nutrition groups, where they count calories together, share recipes for low-fat cakes and cookies, and celebrate weight loss with a hard-earned cheat meal.

But every time Teresa gets on a roll with her exercise and nutrition, another special occasion arises, and Teresa feels obligated to keep up her food-preparing traditions. The gym, the outdoor activities, and the calorie watching are put on the back burner for a week or so as she gears up for the event centered on her traditional tastes: succulent, salty, and sweet. Thus, the cycle of weight gain continues— and so do the weight-related problems.

The 80-100 pounds of excess weight she's been carrying around for close to 30 years has taken a toll on her joints. While Teresa was thinking the countless revolutions on the stationary cardio machines and trekking the trails was doing her body good, all that excess weight as well as her poor gait is causing her body—her "machine"—to break down.

Most disturbing of all is that this lifestyle led to her requiring blood pressure and cholesterol medications for the past 15 years.

Dearest Teresa,

You are an absolutely beautiful, giving person! With this said, consider this letter as your personal intervention— your wake-up call to cool it on the constant celebrating with cherished foods. You are not only celebrating these events because you want to make your family, friends, and students happy. Deeply rooted, you are sticking to these traditions because you yourself desire the succulent, salty, and sweet.

Teresa, you are living to eat, not eating to live.

And you're using these traditions to rationalize treating yourself to your favorite eats and that which comforts you. It's okay to stray from the traditions; think creatively. Con-

Special occasions should be truly special... and only happen occasionally.

sider starting with your students, where maybe you could have a lifelong impact on them by serving healthy options as your new traditions. Think about swapping out all the sugary treats and drinks with things like: unsweetened iced tea with lemon, roasted pumpkin seeds, and seasonal fruits and vegetables. Heck, maybe even coordinate a gardening project as part of a school year craft. Get your kiddos to dig in the dirt; kids love to get dirty!!!

And as far as your family and friends, limit those special occasions. In other words, make them truly "special." There will always be graduations, communions, and picnics, but the line needs to be drawn. While these events should be treated with the recognition they deserve, they can be done without the food-related traditions you've become so accustomed to. And you need to approach your exercise from a different perspective, one that is not so focused on one-dimensional cardio exercise, but rather a comprehensive approach to improving your general, everyday life performance.

Teresa, you're about to retire from your work at the school. But you've still got a life ahead of you—55 is the new 35. It's not too late to transform yourself, and it's actually time to reinvent yourself. Find new traditions that make you happy AND keep you healthy.

AE

CHAPTER 12

Deprivation Donnie

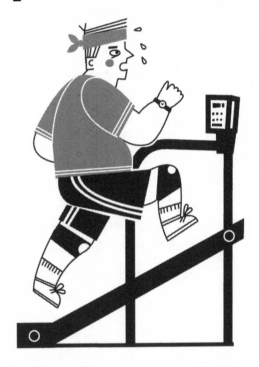

Donnie Daniels is a tough and stubborn son of a gun. Right out of high school, he served a stint in the military, and the boot-camp style mentality has stuck with him ever since. Donnie married Donna when he was in his third year of service, and soon after they had two kids. To no one's surprise, their marriage did not last very long, as they likely married a bit prematurely, and Donnie was just a bitter, opinionated, overly demanding guy to deal with.

Donnie married again in his late 30s, but that marriage

was rocky from the start and only lasted a couple of years as well.

Now in his late 40s, Donnie has been dating Dina for close to seven years. They met while "treadmilling" at their gym when they struck up a conversation about their favorite supplements. They have talked about marriage for some time, but his two failed marriages left a bad taste in Donnie's mouth.

Donnie owns a small and rather successful drywall installation company where he's maintained a staff of five or six guys for over the past 20 years or so. Donnie has his staff perform the on-site installations while he handles the sales end of the business.

When it comes to his physical condition, Donnie is frustrated. At 5'10" and weighing 215 pounds, he's fixated on returning to his military days when he was a lean 165 pounds soaking wet.

Donnie also has multiple issues with his knees (one scoped and one cut) and his shoulders (one scoped, one injected); these issues are mostly a result of his excessive time in the gym.

Donnie attacks his cardio workouts with military-like conviction: headband on, earbuds in, eyes straight ahead, grinding out the revolutions on the elliptical machine or the miles on the treadmill, all with a look of absolute determination—and with a limp gait, unfortunately. But Donnie "knows" what works, as it's worked time and again, and he's absolutely going to sweat his weight off. He performs his cardio day after day, faster and faster, like a hamster on a wheel—sweat pouring off of him, hitting the floor and the machines of the gym that he's been a member of for close to 15 years. He also still walks the neighborhood with a weighted vest three mornings per week and does his 100 push-ups and 100 sit-ups daily before most people arise.

In conjunction with his cardio-based routines, Donnie tries to combat his excess weight with calorie deprivation, where he suppresses his calorie intake to minimal levels for weeks at a time. He eats little to no fat, often skips breakfast, and limits himself to two salads per day.

This tactic usually results in Donnie getting his weight down to 190–195 pounds over and over again, only to climb right back to 215 pounds (over and over again) when he can no longer tolerate the caloric restrictions and excessive exercise and binges for weeks with unfavorable foods such as pizza, hoagies, fast food, and wings. To make matters worse, Donnie has little to no muscle definition whether he's at 190 or 215, as he continues to lose muscle mass with his hard-nosed, cardio-focused training tactics.

Stubborn Donnie never considers hiring a professional performance coach. In his mind, his military basic training days—drive yourself physically and eat only what you need to survive—got him in the best shape of his life. So why would he change what he "knows" works?

In reality Donnie is unhealthy and unhappy, but unfortunately, he knows everything.

Dear Donnie,

Your body is breaking down and will continue to do so until you are willing to tuck your macho tail between your legs and ask a true professional for help. You have to come to the realization that you are not 19 anymore. The human body begins to break down as we age. (This is a scientific fact Donnie; we're all heading to the same place.)

While this is not a death sentence, your training regimen needs to be modified as you age. You need to focus on mobility and corrective exercises so that you can move without feeling crippled. And as far as your fluctuating weight: you need to quit being so darn stubborn and accept your old-school way of undereating and overexercising is not working. Humble yourself Donnie; address your weaknesses rather than hide behind your strengths.

...eat like a man and not like a little rabbit.

In the end, you need to adhere to a proper training program that can help reverse the damage you've inflicted upon yourself with the boot-camp type of approach you've taken for the past 30 years. Hopefully you will begin to eat foods that can be fished, grown, or butchered and approach human performance in a sensible, safe, well-programmed manner. Find a training center whose focus is not on selling memberships to hamsters to run endlessly on wheels, but instead provides a complete, sustainable program that emphasizes mobility and corrective measures and a progressive approach to strength and power.

And last Donnie, eat like an actual man and not like a little rabbit. You can't build a lean, muscular physique on two salads a day!

AE

CHAPTER 13

Super-Fan Sara

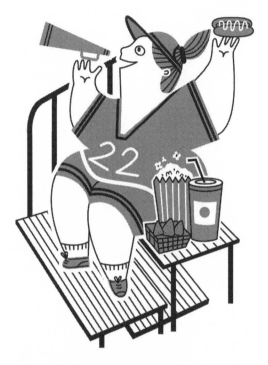

Thirty-three-year-old Sara has worked as a personal assistant for the past 15 years to one of the larger financial executives in the city. Sara is married to her high school sweetheart, Sal, who is an Account Manager for a marketing firm. Sara and Sal identify as die-hard "super fans" of their hometown's major sports teams. The dedicated duo hold season tickets to both their professional hockey team and their perennial power Division 1 basketball team; they also split a ticket package for their city's professional baseball team with two other couples.

Sara and Sal are well known throughout their neighborhood for throwing the ultimate football parties, especially during the playoffs, and their 96-inch projector screen only adds lore to their legendary game-day events.

Outside of work, their lives essentially revolve around gearing up for the next game! They pride themselves on arriving early to the venue and are always sporting their favorite players' regulation jerseys. If they are not tailgating, then they are grabbing a few beers beforehand while they watch any pregame routines. During the games, they eat the traditional super dog, nachos with cheese and bacon bits, the salted soft pretzel, and a couple more beers. They wobble up and down the aisles from their seats (their form of hustle), food in hand each time, anxiously living their lives through these amazing, larger-than-life athletes, all while they become larger than life in their own right.

Their Sunday football parties at home are even more premeditated, and just like the athletes, Sara and Sal have their own pregame routines. Sara wakes early each Sunday to get her special ham barbecue and potato salad recipes going, while Sal mixes up his secret wing sauce formula. After the mainstays are prepared, Sal is off to their membership club store for the super-sized bags of chips and the premium creamy dips, as well as a few cases of beer. Once the game begins, Sara and Sal, along with their neighborhood friends, are well equipped to compete alongside their prized athletes. Though, not truly until halftime are they fully prepared to compete, for this is when the pizza delivery guy shows up to refuel for the second half.

Essentially, Sara and Sal live, breathe, and "eat" their

beloved sports teams.

But despite what appears from the outside looking in as a fun-loving couple whose weeks are filled with friends, parties, and regular "social media moments," behind it all, Sara and Sal are struggling. It's not surprising that they are both quite overweight. Sara tips the scales at 220 pounds at 5'4" tall, and Sal has cracked the 270-pound mark at 5'11". Sara and Sal are in their 30s, and along with the added weight, their physical limitations (due to sheer size) and health-related issues seem to have popped up overnight. Sara's knees throb at night after a day walking the steps of the ballpark, and Sal's doctor prescribed a CPAP machine to combat his sleep apnea, which has worsened as his weight has increased. They both complain of back issues, not to mention they've noticed that even their XXL team jerseys aren't covering up their midsections the way they do for other young couples in the stands. Sadly, Sara and Sal appear to have lived a hard life for their young ages.

They have talked about starting a family, but Sara's doctor suggested she lose a good bit of weight beforehand. Coupled with this matter, they have not taken a really aggressive approach to getting pregnant. Feeling embarrassed by their overweight, nude bodies has put a damper on "game-day activities" in the bedroom, so their sexual interest in each other sits idle on the sidelines. In addition, they're torn about the idea of taking the time to raise a family because they are simply too busy being "super fans."

To combat their excess weight issues, Sara and Sal did what so many do and joined a local 24-hour fitness chain for $10/month (the cost of one beer at the game) with nothing more than the hope of a Hail Mary from their own 20-yard line. The giant fitness chain's marketing campaigns led them to believe that the rows upon rows of hamster wheels and other machines will transform their bodies.

They start off with zest, attacking the elliptical rider like their favorite winger attacks the goal. But of course, they still want to work around the games (and game foods), for they are super fans, after all. After a couple of weeks of little to no weight loss, they decide their schedule is just too busy "in season" to squeeze in workouts, and they'll have to wait until playoffs are over.

Dear Sara and Sal,

Your story resonates on some level with so many of us. Who doesn't like team spirit and the feeling you get when your team wins? But you are both clearly living your lives as idolizing spectators, while your own fitness, performance, health, and body composition head in the exact opposite direction of those you are idolizing. You need to regroup and find purpose beyond living through others. Sara and Sal, you do not need to give up your love of your sports teams altogether, but you've got to find a balance between games and real life (and your relationship to games and gluttony). And a half-hearted stab at fitness is not going to put a dent in your excess weight.

...regroup and find purpose beyond living through others.

Take a serious, well-designed approach to performance training, and keep the gluttonous eating behaviors to special occasions, like the day your team plays in the Super Bowl or Game 7 of the World Series. If not, you will soon be even heavier and will be dealing with much more serious health-related issues. Keep in mind your window for building a family is closing.

It's not too late Sara and Sal, but the time is now!

AE

CHAPTER 14

Witchcraft Willie

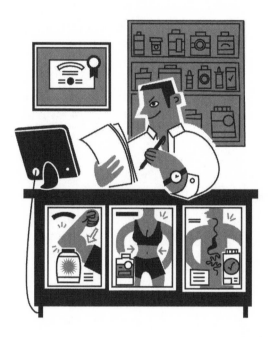

Willie Walters, a charismatic man blessed with a silver tongue and able to sell the fountain of youth to the most vulnerable of the masses, finds himself grappling with profound legal issues and his superstar lifestyle slipping from his grasp. Willie, now in his early 40s, spends much of his time on the phone with his lawyers as they deal with countless fraud scheme legalities.

But not long ago, Willie was flying high with more money to burn than most will see in a lifetime.

Willie had earned his undergraduate and then his doctorate degrees in chemistry by the age of 25. Shortly thereafter, Willie was recruited by a startup nutritional supplement manufacturing company as the head of their research and development team. Willie helped grow the business, developing specially formulated protein powders, bars, vitamin packs, energy tablets, and more. Willie also began to recognize the unbelievable markup on these supplements and how much money could be made.

Eventually Willie left the company, took out a small business loan, and started his own supplement line, using similar formulas he helped develop at his old company. But he decided to go beyond the commonly available supplements and began to explore new lines of extracts from remote parts of the world. He traveled to rain forests, jungles, high-altitude mountain terrains, and small exotic islands in search of ingredients for the fountain of youth. Willie recorded many of these excursions and created a rather significant following on multiple social media platforms.

By 30, Willie opened his first storefront practice, *Dr. Willie's Wellness and Healing Center.* And since he had a PhD in Chemistry, he didn't feel the need to correct clients who assumed he was a medical doctor. With that credential, he felt comfortable charging premium fees for one-on-one "health" consultations, either with himself or with one of his assistants. Usually, his consultations led to orders for extensive (and expensive) blood work panels, which he then would match up with one or more of his specially formulated products to counter any of the slightest of imbalances.

His typical client was the vulnerable type—middle-aged, usually overweight or obese, with chronic pain and inflammation, low testosterone, metabolic syndrome, and/or chronic fatigue.

Willie was so convincing in his abilities to cure that he could convince a 50-year-old man to buy a unicorn-hoof extract that promised a sex drive five times higher than what he experienced in his teens and 20s. Willie was not only a "doctor," but he was charming to boot.

"Dr." Willie's specialty was *gut health,* and he formulated a proprietary rich blend of probiotics and greens, known as U-Gut-This Greens, for weight loss and chronic inflammation. Willie was so aggressive in his marketing that he even began touting that his products and programs could cure certain forms of cancer. Unhealthy folks were lining up to become "Dr." Willie's patients, and they had no reservations about signing up for all the products Willie recommended. Willie's vision was working perfectly, as his key business strategy was having his patients sign a two-year contract where their checking accounts would be tagged with fees ranging from $150 to $600 per month.

"Dr." Willie took to sponsored ads on social media and local TV spots to promote his business, and his charisma helped his client base grow more so than any success stories. He opened a few more wellness centers, and soon Willie's fortune grew, too. Willie had hundreds upon hundreds of clients and was making well over a million dollars per year with his product lines and consulting business. By the time he reached 40, his lifestyle included a $100,000 sports car, a large house, and a mountain retreat. He dated numerous women, many of whom were clients under his care.

Ironically, Willie himself frequently came down with colds and always seemed to have a chronic inflammation ailment. Yet he ate very little whole food, often adhering to extended periods of intermittent fasting; and what he did consume were mostly his own specially engineered supplements.

Willie was thin and looked great in his custom suits. But in reality, he had very little muscle mass on his body and was quite soft and mushy. Willie seemed to have the material world by the tail, yet he was feeling unhealthy, and somewhere deep down inside, he knew he was a fraud.

Things got even worse for Willie. It turns out that a client with advanced cancer, who he had been treating for some time, recently passed away. During his time with her, Willie originally ordered a blood profile panel, and after assessing the report, he set her up on a multitude of supplements promising to cure this nasty disease "naturally."

Unfortunately, this woman's cancer progressed, and eventually she lost her battle. After her death, the woman's family learned of and was outraged by the unsubstantiated claims Willie promised their mother, and they filed suit for wrongful death. Once this hit the news, other patients of Willie's filed claims, stating the two-year contract they signed was unreasonable. Other patients whose health had deteriorated because they were influenced to leave their medical doctor's advice for Willie's "natural" cures also came forward. To add salt to the wound, Willie also got sued by his original employer, for Willie violated a non-compete and nondisclosure contract he had signed when he started his employment there.

Dear Willie,

You have preyed on the weak and vulnerable, and now you are clearly paying the price with your personal health and finances. You've chosen to take the shortcuts yourself, and you've spread these shortcuts to the masses in a money-making scheme, so you'll need to pay your dues.

But Willie, you have the chance to do something special. What if you took these hard lessons and rebranded yourself as the reformed guy who will help the masses transform the correct way, and take up battle against those of the wicked selling witchcraft potions? You could teach the vulnerable masses that supplements have their place, as many folks have nutrient deficiencies and other health issues that truly require supplementation. But when the witchcraft potions of those money mongers promise the fountain of youth, the beautiful bodies, to cure all pain and suffering, to reverse horrible diseases such as cancer, teach the masses to pay no mind.

Karma is truly a bitch, Willie

Willie, reevaluate your life's values. And implement proper training, nutrition (through real food that can be fished, grown, or butchered), and stress reduction into your own life for both your own personal health and for those whom you could lead by example.

Karma is truly a bitch, Willie—humbly lead others.

AE

CHAPTER 15

All-Business Alison

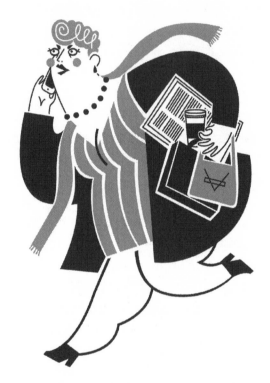

Alison is a 52-year-old attorney and a partner at one of the city's largest firms. Alison is used to winning in both the courtroom and the business world, at all costs. Both her strong personality and intense competitiveness in the courtroom spill over into her personal life's persona. Alison expects perfection from those who provide service to her, such as waiters, waitresses, and valet attendants, and she never hesitates to remind them that she's a partner in a law firm. Her girlfriends look to Alison to pick the restaurant, plan the girls' getaway weekends, and choose the next read for the Book Club; few dare to debate her choices. Alison's twin girls are out of college and have jobs in other cities. When they do come to town, it's usually a quick visit that's scheduled around their mom's appointments. The remainder of their weekend is spent with their dad, Alison's ex-husband, Allen. The two divorced while the girls were in high school, citing irreconcilable differences. There are always two sides to every story, but most people close to the couple believe Alison's frequency of putting her work before her family played a major role in the split.

Alison has essentially won in her career for years on end, but the one adversary she has yet to defeat is her weight. She has struggled with her size as early as her late teen years, but particularly more so since her late 20s, after the birth of her twins and the high demands of her illustrious career really kicked into gear. While she has been able to lose *some* weight quite a few times over the past 20 years, as well as hide much of her excess weight with her custom-fit wardrobe, she is now at an all-time high, cracking the 200-pound mark for the first time. Also, as of late, she's finding it harder and harder to look at herself in the mirror while undressed.

She knows she's losing her battle with her weight, which is causing her much angst and despair. So she's decided to defeat it…since winning is what she does.

Through years of litigation, Alison has become very used to dealing with the most sought-after experts in her field, and she sticks to that rule when it comes to her world outside of business, including fitness. She joined an elite gym across town from her office because she heard it employs the most well-known (and expensive) trainers in the area. But she makes it clear to those trainers that her work comes before her workout. Alison arrives right at the start of the appointment and not a minute before, keeping her phone close by on the gym floor and stopping a few times during the session to take very important litigation calls, as well as answer e-mails in between sets. When the training hour is up, she exits right away, often to take a conference call in the parking lot.

On weekends, she attends classes at a premier Yoga and Pilates studio, where she again takes her phone in—on silent, of course—and handles her text messages and e-mails from her child's pose. Alison wonders, "Who in the world has time to just lay there and breathe when decisions need to be made?"

Alison's competitive and "only the best" nature complicates and undermines her relationship with food, too. When the topic of food comes up, whether with friends, her personal trainer, or her yoga instructor, she speaks with conviction and deflects her own weight struggles at hand. She power shops at a trendy organic grocery store near her home in the city, hits the local farmers market every Sunday morning, grabs her coffee from the environmentally aware national brew house each morning, and picks up salads from the local health-conscious deli next to her office each day for lunch. Yet she sabotages her efforts as that coffee turns into a latte and croissant, and her salad is piled with cheese she thinks is best because it's produced from grass-fed cows and includes gluten-free croutons and loads of "healthy" oils.

She snacks on organic kale chips and dips, as well as non-GMO protein bars, and after a long day of deals and deadlines, she unwinds with a few glasses of red wine before dinner to take the edge off of another hectic day. In her mind, wine is high in antioxidants, after all.

When it comes to dinner, as far as Alison is concerned she is simply too busy with her important job to prepare meals. So dinner is generally alone in her three-story custom-built, interior-designed condo overlooking the city, with a meal she heats up from a local health food preparation and delivery service that delivers a week's worth of prepared, precooked, microwavable "healthy" meals to her doorstep. In the late evening, when going over her files for the next morning's court appearance, she has a large bowl of low-sugar, low-fat, low-everything frozen yogurt with a few tablespoons of local honey and a chunk or two of "highly beneficial" dark chocolate.

Alison appears to be full of conviction, yet behind closed doors, her excess weight, the loss of her marriage, the absence of a significant other at her age, and her kids being all grown up and in other cities has taken its toll. Despite her occasional gatherings with girlfriends, she's extremely lonely and sad, and wonders how she can be so successful in the business world and have so much clout, not to mention her material wealth, yet her own relationships and physical appearance are a wreck. Bottom line: this winning attorney feels absolutely defeated.

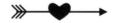

Dear Alison,

You have so much, yet so little. You're a partner at your law firm—congratulations! That had to have taken quite the commitment. But it also sounds like it has come at a cost. How much money do you need? How powerful do you need to feel?

You absolutely have to commit to stepping away from the constant connectivity of work and reflect on what really matters: your own health and happiness. You also need to let down your guard and accept that you need help with understanding how food plays a significant role in the success and failure of weight control.

You're fooling yourself if you think your "organic, natural" approach to food is "natural"—hipster lattes, mounds of cheese, dark chocolate, croissants, red wine, kale chips, and so on. And protein bars (aka glorified candy bars), too? Really, Alison? Day in and day out you essentially sabotage almost everything you consume. Drink your coffee black! Skip the croissants, mounds of cheese and oils, and limit the wine and dark chocolate to special occasions!

Alison— you're not all that important.

Also, accept that maybe the most "well-known" trainers aren't necessarily the most beneficial. Commit to a proper training and nutrition program. Find a coach who can program correctly, where you train sensibly and sustainably. Finally, take time to shop and prepare your own darn meals.

Life is so short Alison, and you're still young with a full life ahead: friendships, your daughters' marriages, grandchildren, and possibly a new romance. Commit to working less and sleeping more so you don't look and feel so rundown. Turn off your phone Alison—you're not all that important. You're 52 years old. This is not a death sentence. It's time to humble yourself and get your "personal groove" back!

Woman up, Alison!

AE

CHAPTER 16

Super-Fly Sonny

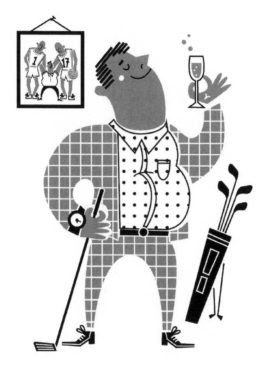

Sonny is simply THE man. He can definitely be called "self-made," as he owns a franchise department store where he started as an eager stock boy at age 17 and quickly worked his way up through management. He earned the utmost trust of the store's original owner, who took Sonny under his wing and taught him everything he knew in the years to follow. When the time was right, Sonny got a loan from the bank and bought the store from the retiring owner. After a few more years of grinding away and a couple of sweet business decisions, Sonny's store was doing really well. He started making the kind of money that 17-year-old "stock boy Sonny" had only dreamed of.

Early in his booming business career, Sonny married Sherry, a woman he met at a trendy nightclub a few months after he bought his business. After a whirlwind romance and six-month engagement, they threw a monster wedding at one of the city's finest venues.

As Sonny's business grew, so did his and Sherry's thirst for material goods and being in the limelight. Sonny began wearing only the finest custom-made suits, and the majority of Sherry's wardrobe was bought on one of her many quick shopping trips to New York. He and Sherry bought a million-dollar home, joined an exclusive country club, and had connections that landed them front-row season tickets to the local collegiate and professional sports teams' games.

Sonny and Sherry became known as the local celebrity couple that knew how to party. They developed quite the reputation at their country club as the duo that closed the place down night after night with their wild drinking. Their publicly intoxicated behavior at sports venues created quite a buzz around town. Sonny also started doing TV spots for his business that added to his local celebrity status.

Sonny is always where the action is. If golf pros are in town, he's available to sponsor and play with them for a practice round. If the football team is hosting a fundraiser, Sonny figures out a way to buddy up and hang with the popular jocks at the event. And Sonny is almost always the life of the event, drinking up a storm and cracking jokes with "the boys," leaving them in stitches. As a matter of fact, Sonny's office is full of pictures of himself (and occasionally Sherry) with local sports and entertainment celebrities: his own personal "Wall of Fame."

Sonny is liked by everyone. He's charming, a big tipper, and always the best dressed with the finest jewelry. What's not to like?

But deep down, Sonny is hurting. He and his wife have no children—which was their decision as they share the opinion that kids are too time-consuming—and as he's now in his late 40s, he's beginning to regret this decision. He can't stand the way his body feels and performs: his joints ache, his mobility is that of a tin man, and when it comes to the passion of his life, golf, he's barely strong enough to hit his drives past the ladies' tee.

Furthermore, his physique is a disaster, where only his custom-fit suits, shirts, sport coats and slacks hide his boob-like chest and his four inches of belly fat hanging over his waistband.

Sherry, who at one time was his right-hand gal at all the events, has become insatiable in that she cannot buy enough consumer goods to make herself happy. She meets up with her group of friends to play golf a couple times a week, always finishing the round with a bottle of wine and a cheese plate. She joins another group of friends at her paddle tennis club two times a week as well, grabbing lunch afterward, which includes more wine and cheese as well as some tasty appetizers from the bar.

Sherry's not happy with what she sees in the mirror either, as her once young, tight body is hidden somewhere under the 30 pounds of fat she's put on over the last few years. Worse, she's become jealous of Sonny's iconic image and now resents his success.

In recent years, they've grown apart and seem more like "housemates" than husband and wife as they rattle around in their large home, barely seeing each other between her golf, paddle, and social outings and his "celebrity" obligations.

Despite the distance between them, Sonny and Sherry continue on their path of fancy dining, concerts, and celebrity gatherings, all with heavy drinking. The framed celebrity and sports figure photos on Sonny's office walls continue to grow.

But with each picture, the athletes and celebrities appear to become more physically fit, attractive, and younger, and Sonny and Sherry appear to be aging, and their bodies seem to be swelling at a rapid rate.

Dear Sonny,

Your Wall of Fame tells a profound and sad story of the rise and decline of your Super-Fly Sonny persona and your once sexy wife, Sherry. You've selfishly lived in the spotlight long enough, and if you don't wake up and make a major change in your partying lifestyles, one of you may, well...one of you may not wake up.

Yes, you passed on having your own children. But goodness, with your successes you could help so many youth organizations in need. And not just with your money, but with your precious time. Reconnect with one another and help these children or even a specific child. Turn back the clock and live that life you passed on, now.

And as far as your physical health, you two absolutely

have to begin training and eating correctly. *A lifelong journey to improved health, performance, and body composition can be accomplished through a properly designed nutrition and training program, along with humility, purpose, and faith.*

Sonny, I beg you to see the light before it's too late.

Discontinue living the American success story to unquenchable levels. No matter the material conquests, your well-being simply cannot be bought. It must be earned.

Sonny, I beg you to see the light before it's too late.

AE

CHAPTER 17

Hunter Hugh

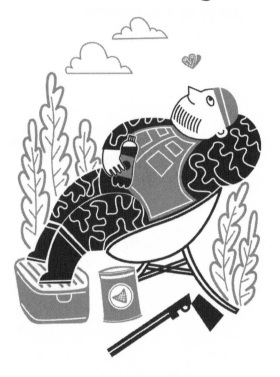

Hugh is the quintessential manly man. He is married to Holly, his grade school sweetheart, and they have three young boys. Hugh grew up with a rugged, loving father who taught him at an early age how to live off and respect the land by hunting and fishing. Hugh has been a die-hard outdoors man ever since, and plans to pass down his hunting traditions to all three of his boys. Hugh does not hunt for sport; rather he hunts to supply food for his family. His typical hunts are for deer, elk, turkey, and pheasant.

Hugh has always been a pretty big guy. At 6'3" tall and weighing in at a lean 210 pounds, he was a natural and a star defensive end for his high school football team. His father was a big man as well, standing 6'4" tall and weighing a lean 215 pounds throughout his early years of fatherhood.

These days, Hugh's tradition of hunting includes three or four trips to the same cabin he grew up going to with his father and his father's friends. But now, Hugh goes with a group of his own friends who he's been hunting with since his early teens. Hugh also goes on a couple of fishing trips with his buddies: trout fishing in the spring up in the mountains, deep-sea fishing in the summer, and salmon fishing up North in the late summer. In addition, Hugh is involved heavily in his sportsmen's club and participates in multiple pheasant hunts throughout the year.

Hugh is considered by most to be a very grounded man. His family doesn't own luxury cars or live in a large, suburban home in a neighborhood plan. However, he and Holly have splurged on "his and hers" platinum pickup trucks with front vanity plates: one for Hugh that reads "WEHUNT4FOOD" and one for Holly that reads "WEFISH4FOOD," as well as the large post-and-beam home they built on a four-acre lot on the outskirts of a much sought-after school district. Hugh and Holly have strong faith, attend church in the front pew every Sunday, and volunteer at their church's yearly fundraisers (fish fries, spaghetti dinners, pancake breakfasts, and more), and they each often lead their church's men's and women's Bible study sessions throughout the year.

Though Hugh is humble in many ways, he takes pride and actually likes to brag about his ability to provide his family with a portion of their food intake throughout the year. He's also proud that he processes much of his own meat in a little man cave that he calls his "barn and butchery." He likes to talk about his family's two additional freezer chests full of elk and venison steaks, chops, roasts, and ground meat, as well as frozen turkeys, pheasant, and fish.

Hugh and Holly, now in their late 30s, appear to possess quite the little slice of Americana. But all is not perfect. In recent years, Hugh has ballooned up to a whopping 290 pounds, and his wife Holly has grown to 210 pounds. This is quite a change from when she was in high school, where at 5'5" and 130 pounds, she co-captained the cheerleading squad, rooting for her future husband, Hugh. In addition, Hugh is on multiple medications for his heart, and has significant orthopedic issues with his feet. Holly has had one knee partially replaced, and is now looking at hip surgery. She's not happy with how she looks or feels and is not sure how and when all this happened to her once athletic frame. On top of this, their three boys, who to no one's surprise are avid hunters and fishermen, are all overweight as well.

Hugh and his buddies like to get together a half-dozen times each year for long weekends where they hunt and fish for their families. But they also get together to live it up a bit. They enjoy case after case of beer in the afternoons and evenings, and they cook up all of their special recipe foods from previous hunts, like hot sausage, bratwurst, bacon, fried turkey, and pheasant in peanut oil, and heavily battered and fried fish. The hot sausage and bratwurst taste best on the thick buns they picked up (along with the rich sauce and fried onions and peppers); the pan-fried bacon is a must with the pan-fried eggs as well as thick pancakes with butter and maple syrup; the succulent fried turkey and pheasant make perfect sandwiches (along with cheese, mayo, and some leftover bacon); and the long-awaited breaded and deep-fried fish go great with potato salad and coleslaw.

And those pheasant hunts at the sportsmen's club are more than Hugh providing for his family. Hugh's morning hunt turns into an afternoon full of beers, cheers, and manly bowls of thick, sausage-filled chili topped with mounds of cheese and served with crackers and rolls.

Hugh's habits at home are not all that different. His freezer is packed with his special hot sausage and bratwurst recipes that are full of sugar, salt, and more, and his family finds themselves eating these foods quite often. They also frequently take the lean ground venison and pan fry it before adding it to their spaghetti sauce recipe that goes on top of linguine pasta noodles and served with Parmesan cheese and fresh Italian bread. For Hugh and Holly there will be a few glasses of red wine, and for the boys, homemade sweetened iced tea. In addition, they also take their lean meats that Hugh so ruggedly hunted for and make things like tacos, burritos, meatloaf, and more. And Hugh's fridge in his man cave is always filled with his favorite seasonal beers.

The gluttonous behavior continues even at their Bible study sessions, as they always include cookies, doughnuts, or other pastries (usually at the direction of Hugh and Holly), and those volunteer fundraiser nights are essentially a license to eat.

Culminating these poor habits, Hugh works as a chief estimator for a high revenue-producing national contractor, where days can be long and often turn into nights when bids are due. The stress on Hugh takes its toll on him, but in order to allow Holly to be a stay-at-home mom and to keep up with the platinum truck payments and the large mortgage and real estate taxes on the home and the property in that exclusive school district, Hugh has no choice but to keep grinding.

So despite Hugh's nature-filled hunting and fishing pastimes and the couple's grounded, faith-filled lifestyle, Hugh, Holly, and their boys are not the lean machines that nature intended for those who live to hunt or fish. They are paying the price for ignoring that which could be theirs. Holly is unhappy and embarrassed with the extra weight she's gained, and her body is breaking down as a result. Hugh is quite unhealthy and stressed and has his own orthopedic issues directly related to weight. Their three boys are already having some emotional issues related to their weight among their peers, particularly at gym class and in the locker room.

Dear Hugh,

The purpose of my letter to you is not to single out any one specific population like hunters or their families. The aim is to emphasize how you and your family, along with so many of us, no matter socio-economics or cultures, rationalize our actual food intake. You and your family are falling victim to the need for the "succulent, salty, and sweet," and are living life to eat.

Hugh, you are such an avid hunter and outdoorsman. The animals you hunt and fish provide so many lean foods at your fingertips. You don't need hot sausage or bratwurst, nor do you need tacos, cheesy and greasy spaghetti, or burritos.

Consider grilling (not frying) those elk and venison chops and serving them with a plain baked potato and steamed veggies. Poach those fish fillets with green and red peppers and onions and serve them on a bed of steamed jasmine rice. Roast the turkey and pheasant and serve it with boiled quinoa and blanched green beans. And as for the Bible study fare, how about a vegetable tray rather than your usual pastries? Live life truly the way you proclaim with those vanity plates and your respect for Mother Nature. Downsize those pickups, man, and reduce that stress level.

A heart attack does you no good and leaves your family without a father.

A heart attack does you no good and leaves your family without the father figure you had. Do this for your marriage, do this for your children, and do this for a long, healthy, and happy future.

AE

CHAPTER 18

Farmer Frank

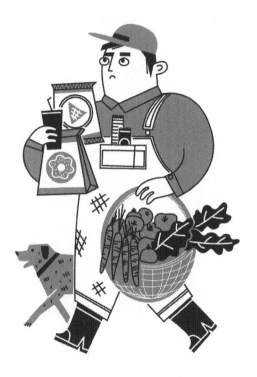

In 1988, 9-year-old Frank was following right in his family's footsteps as a fifth-generation farmer in training. He came from a long line of rugged, hardworking, American men and women who lived the lives depicted in classic midwestern imagery. They were lean and muscular farmers whose days were spent plowing, digging, planting, baling, and tending to livestock. His family literally lived off their land and their farm for generations. They raised chickens for eggs and meat, tended to cattle for beef, trolled ponds and streams for fish, and had access to acres upon acres of fresh food crops. What they could not harvest or produce on their own, they bartered with neighboring farms.

As a by-product of their hardy, manual-intense lifestyle and livelihoods, Frank's family members were generally very lean and muscular. As a teen, it was clear that Frank had inherited the same farmer physique since he lived and breathed this farming life. Frank embraced his rural upbringing and planned to make farming his career and one day take charge of his family's enterprise. Slated to be the first in his family to attend college, Frank would earn his education at his home state university that was known for its top-notch Agriculture Department. The stage was set for Frank's healthy, happy life of farming.

While attending college, he met his future wife Fran, who was also from a small town and studying agriculture. It was pretty much love at first sight. They were well suited for each other as Frank and Fran both enjoyed the peace, tranquility, and self-sustainability of the farming lifestyle and also shared a bad taste for the pace of bigger cities.

The summer after their college graduation, Fran moved to Frank's hometown following their romantic, barn-style wedding, and shortly thereafter, the two agriculture degree grads would take over Frank's family farm. It was official—the young, steadfast newlyweds were a full-time, fifth-generation farming couple.

In their early-to-mid 20s, the couple arose together before 5:00 a.m. every day to tend to the livestock—loading bales of hay and sacks of grain into the paddocks, emptying and filling water troughs, and shoveling bucket after bucket of manure. Fran worked right alongside her studly husband Frank in the early years. But once their family began to grow, Fran spent a little less time in the fields, as she had her hands full inside the house. It wasn't long after their little ones could walk that they, too, were given chores they could manage, like feeding and cleaning up after the chickens, collecting fruits and vegetables, and other manageable tasks throughout the day.

From a nutrition standpoint, young Frank, Fran and the kids adhered to the typical "Mother Nature" meals of yesteryear. The adults began their days with a good ole' cup of black coffee, while the children drank milk or tea. After their early morning chores, they enjoyed a couple of small but satisfying portions of farm-raised eggs from the chicken house, a slice of farm-raised ham, a piece of Fran's freshly baked loaf of grain bread, and a wedge or two of a succulent tomato picked straight from the vine. After more work on the farm, they broke for a lunch of fresh produce and whole grains that were harvested on their very own land, with perhaps a slice or two of beef from the cattle that was butchered from the back fifty earlier in the summer and grilled the night before. In between meals, snacks consisted of the taste of a carrot plucked fresh from the dirt or the berries pulled directly from the berry patch. Again after more hard work during the afternoon in the heavy sun, Frank, Fran, and their young children would stop and gather together for a traditional family dinner that was centered around foods like a whole roasted chicken raised on the farm paired with vegetables harvested off their land and often complemented with home-grown baked potatoes and a garden-fresh salad packed with greens and cucumbers. Dessert was frequently some tasty homemade applesauce made from the apples in the orchard.

Frank and Fran's lifestyle early in their marriage was much like that of the generations that preceded them. They were lean, fit, and grounded folk. But unfortunately for Frank's young family, they were part of the generation that experienced a significant change in the culture and the huge boom of processed foods and "convenience eating." This boom hit the big cities years ago, but most recently made its way into small-town USA. Coincidentally, Frank's family, like many other farming families at that time, started to "grow" in circumference at the same time this processed phenomenon hit full stride.

Flash forward to the present: Frank and Fran are now approaching 40 and with four teenage kids, have completely different eating habits than their twentysomething selves. Breakfast often starts with the drive-through doughnut shop that replaced the farmer's market in town years ago, where Frank generally snags a dozen iced pastries each morning before chores start. He grabs coffee (or more likely calorie-laden mocha lattes) for the family from the national coffee chain that opened quite a few locations not far from their farm.

Snacks and drinks have changed dramatically as well, and Frank finds it much more efficient to have a pack of cheese crackers or maybe a scrumptious candy bar or two in his overalls while he manages the hired farm workers. This way he doesn't have to take a break for a snack. And to quench his and his family's thirst, the old-time farmers' pitchers once filled with clean, fresh, cold well water have now been replaced with convenient and easy-to-grab energy drinks or cans of soda, loaded with extra unnecessary chemicals and calories.

Lunches for the family are now most often sandwiches made of maple honey chipped ham lunch meat on delicious, processed white bread and topped with a few tablespoons of creamy mayonnaise, along with some chips and a soda— all from the local convenience store.

Dinner has evolved a "tiny" bit as well; they still eat chicken, but now the chickens are breaded and fried, served with mashed potatoes with heavy cream and butter and topped with gravy, with a side of creamy coleslaw. The meal is finished off with some store-bought apple pie and served with a couple scoops of vanilla ice cream with chocolate and peanut butter chips in it.

In the late evening, Frank and family sit down after a long day of farming and catch up on their favorite shows on their high-def, flat-screen TV for a couple of hours. If their teenagers are around, they're on their own devices: smartphones, laptops, etc. It's during this newfound "family bonding time" that the family treat themselves to another reheated piece of that apple pie with another scoop or two of that ice cream while taking in the shows. Frank's family members do not sleep as much as they used to. Even though they still begin their farming day at 5:00 a.m., squeezing in a couple hours of TV each night and catching up on e-mails and social media pushes their bedtimes later in the evening.

Present-day Frank and Fran are both experiencing health problems. Frank is turning 40 years old in six months and has become very unhappy with himself. When he married Fran, he was a lean 175 pounds, and standing at 6'2" tall, he was nothing but muscle back then. Now he tips the scales at 250-plus pounds, his knees are shot (literally, as he has to get injections twice a year until he needs to have them replaced), he takes blood pressure medication, and his low back is a wreck. Frank finds himself often looking at their framed wedding day picture and wondering how this transformation has taken place in what seems like just yesterday.

Fran just turned 39 and has recently been diagnosed with Type 2 diabetes. She is 70 pounds heavier than when she and Frank married in their early 20s, and she's lost a tremendous amount of confidence. She lives on a beautiful farm in a custom-built country-style home and is surrounded by nature and serenity. Yet she is embarrassed by the way she looks and upset with herself because of the number of medications she is taking. To make matters worse, the small, lucrative market Frank built as an addition to one of their barns for Fran to sell all their fresh meat and produce "weighs" on her heavily, as she's particularly embarrassed to be overweight while she sells all of these so-called "Farm-Fresh" health foods.

Last, adding salt to their wounds, they're both distraught that the youngest two of their four children (two girls) are quite overweight and are having social issues in high school as a result of their unhappiness with their appearance; they've received taunting texts, e-mails, and social media insults on their smartphones. The double icing on the cake (pun intended) is that neither Frank nor Fran has any remote urge to connect with the other's intimate or sexual needs, wants, and desires.

Dear Frank,

You are surrounded by Mother Nature and the nutrient-rich foods she provides. Generations before you lived a simple life of hard work and providing for themselves. You, yourself raise cattle and poultry and grow produce to make a living, and quite honestly, what an admirable way to pass on life lessons to your family and generations to come.

But for goodness' sake, man, you are living the farming life of a hypocrite! You are surrounded like few others with Mother Nature's bountiful offerings, yet you and your family have still fallen victim to the seduction of the "salty, savory, and sweet" epidemic, all wrapped up in a convenient package.

Frank, you have to wake up to see the direct relationship between your family's drastic change of eating habits over the last two decades and the deterioration of their health, confidence, and appearance.

Man, you've got to rein this in. You're tough, you're disciplined—you're a badass, American farmer! But you're displaying weakness and ignorance not only to yourself, but your beloved family as well, and as a parent, you need to lead by example.

Get back to your roots, Frank. What worked as recently as a couple of decades ago is the answer to your issues. It's not complicated. Get back to that simplicity of eating what can be fished, grown, and butchered in its unadulterated state. Limit the television and those damn smartphones that your entire family is addicted to. Get back to the humble man raising a humble family that does not need to live their lives through others.

Demand more sleep for you and your entire family, Frank. You are not a young pup any longer who can run on adrenaline. Your body is breaking down from inadequate rest and too much weight on your body while living a demanding physical lifestyle over the years. Lastly, you're turning 40, and you've put a lot of manual labor stress on your body without truly performing any quality service. You need to get involved in a physical performance training program to help you with mobility, corrective movements, and general fitness so that you can continue to live an active career without such a high risk of injury.

Frank, you have one huge advantage over your ancestors: science! Where many of their bodies broke down in their later years as a result of excessive labor and not a remote thought of an exercise program or adequate recovery, you and your family have the wisdom of proper, present-day training on your side. Today's science tells us

Wake up Frank, Mother Nature's bountiful offerings surround you.

that the body needs to recover, and we also understand the support mechanisms of the body that need to be trained. Get your entire family training sustainably!

Make these changes for your wife; help her feel beautiful again, and bring a fire back to your marriage for years to come. Make these changes for your children; help them develop a healthy self-image and well-being, so they can conquer their worlds with confidence.

AE

Vegetarian Virginia

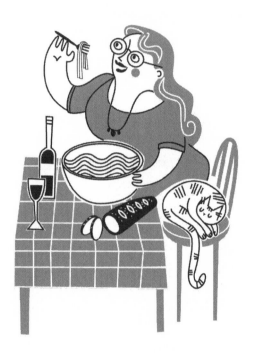

irginia is a 37-year-old mother of one beautiful little 8-year-old girl, Vivian and wife to 38-year-old Vince, and she loves to joke with friends and family that she reeled in an older man. Virginia and her family live on a small cul-de-sac in a cute two-story cedar home with their two Golden Retrievers and their lovable little kitty. Virginia has worked as a filing clerk for the city's tax department at their main headquarters downtown since graduating from college, and Vince works for the township they live in as an assistant code officer and also runs the township animal shelter and its fundraising initiatives.

Virginia has been an animal lover her entire life, seemingly always having a puppy or kitten at one time or another throughout her childhood. When she met Vince and found out his occupation, she knew she had found her soulmate. Ever since their Vivian was old enough to walk, the entire family has volunteered at the animal shelter every Saturday morning.

However, the animal-loving, 5'3" Virginia has not been in love with her body since her midteens. Her weight has fluctuated over the years; it's been as low as 135 pounds when she married Vince ten years ago and as high as her current weight of 185 pounds. Virginia is uncomfortable with her size and her appearance and tries diligently to keep a slimmer figure as she so desperately feels she's letting her husband down. She's also unhappy that her joints ache, and she's feeling a bit run-down and down in the dumps more often than not.

Virginia became a vegetarian in her late teens after a film documentary she saw led her to do a research project in her second year of college, which opened her eyes about the mass production of cattle and poultry. Coupled with her innate love for animals and the fact her weight hit an all-time high—165 pounds after her freshman year and a bit of excess partying—Virginia felt she found her true calling in relation to food.

The then-college student Virginia immediately began to see her weight drop as she cut out the late-night pepperoni pizzas, the morning sausage biscuits, and the afternoon hamburgers and fries. Virginia ate toast with jam for breakfast, salads for lunch and dinner, and avoided going out with friends, as she knew the night would end up with some sort of feast that didn't match her vegetarian lifestyle. Virginia also added running into her schedule, getting in a three-mile run after dinner three or four times a week. In no time, Virginia dropped 20 pounds (almost unheard of for a college student) and was elated with her accomplishments and her appearance.

For Virginia, her rigorous commitment to vegetarianism unfortunately meant a less-than-exciting social life, especially for a college kid. To avoid the food temptations, she was rarely hanging with her girlfriends, nor was she meeting any boys. So after a couple months of strict adherence to her vegetarian lifestyle, Virginia let down her guard and started going out with friends, where she realized she *could* still have that late-night pizza—she just needed to get it with cheese and veggies instead of pepperoni or sausage. And beer is vegetarian, right? Virginia was enjoying life again, meeting people and feeling like a social butterfly, but not too long after, she found her weight back up to where it started.

As Virginia battled her weight over the years, she immersed herself in online research on "superfoods" and supplements that would assist her in her vegetarian lifestyle as well as her hopes of maintaining a slim figure. There were times when she'd buckle down and focus on weight loss, like the six months leading up to her wedding where she stuck to a very low-calorie diet and ran every day to get her weight to that magical 135 pounds for her big day! However, that was the last time she's seen anything remotely close to that weight.

Fast-forward to the present and a look into the daily nutrition of the now 185-pound Virginia. For breakfast, she has a protein smoothie concocted of mocha-flavored vegetable protein powder mixed with 12 ounces of almond milk, 1/4 cup of organic oats, omega-3 capsules, ground coconut, pomegranate, and a banana. She pairs her "potion" with a soy protein-enriched slice of toast with organic jam.

Each morning when she gets into town, she hits her favorite trendy coffee shop for her special latte and generally goes with the seasonal offering, such as the pumpkin spice, triple-whipped latte. She can't wait to get to work and enjoy this treat with her vanilla protein bar enriched with soy nuggets. Lunchtime means she hits up a hipster cafe for tapioca flour-crusted quinoa with guacamole and flax seeds, topped with a Mediterranean vinaigrette dressing and served with a gluten-free roll. For her long ride home, she's packed another protein bar; this time it's a Double-Dark Delight to satisfy her "chocolate fix." For dinner, Virginia prepares a tasty pasta dish of boiled linguini noodles, browned and baked meatballs made of tofu, breadcrumbs, sautéed onions and peppers, and a touch of salt and sugar with marinara sauce. This delicious meal is then served with mozzarella cheese bread (Vivian's favorite) and a glass of red wine with her hubby, Vince. Late in the evening, Virginia likes to be sure she gets her protein in before she sleeps, so she has a couple of tablespoons of cashew butter and an 8 oz. glass of vanilla-flavored almond milk.

In an attempt to shed pounds, Virginia turns to her tried-and-true exercise partner: running. She periodically starts up a running campaign and hits the local running trails a few times a week. She couples her campaign with an all-out effort to cut calories to below 1,000 per day, carefully logging everything she eats, and she's happy seeing the scale numbers start to drop. However, after a few weeks of it, she gives up because her knee pain flares up, the calorie suppression is too challenging, and the logging becomes burdensome. She falls back into her old patterns, and the cycle continues.

Dear Virginia,

Your commitment to your vegetarian lifestyle is admirable, but you are simply sabotaging your approach to food and ultimately your weight and your health. You have somehow justified hundreds upon hundreds of so-called "healthy" excess calories to your vegetarian lifestyle.

It's no surprise that you're struggling with your weight. When you've attempted to lose weight by dropping your calorie intake and increasing your exercise (eating very little and adding running into your routine), yes, you've lost weight! But your body most likely lost a good bit of muscle and with that, a good bit of metabolism. So as soon as you let your guard down and eat more, your weight shoots back up because your metabolism is suppressed.

Rather than tainting the nutrient-rich foods you consume with excess calories the way you do, why not prepare and consume them plainly and simply? Your breakfast could be as basic as a bowl of steel-cut oats topped with fresh raspberries served alongside an unsweetened scoop of a vegetable protein supplement. Rather than your glorified candy bar (i.e., your protein bar) you could simply have an apple and a half an ounce of walnuts. For lunch, that quinoa is a great idea, but could it simply be a boiled bowl of quinoa with added roasted veggies and topped with a couple hard-boiled eggs, adding sea salt and pepper for flavoring. Replace that chocolate bar you have on your ride home with another piece of fruit and a pinch of flax seeds. For dinner, how about grilling a block of plain tofu with basic seasonings and serving it on top of a bed of wild rice pilaf and grilled broccoli and red pepper, with a side salad of mixed greens tossed with an olive oil vinaigrette? And lastly, for that late-night evening snack: sure, your cashew butter is okay because it has a small amount of protein, but keep it to a teaspoon, as it also has a high fat content, and keep that "unsweetened" almond milk to 4 oz. or so.

You're sabotaging your vegetarian lifestyle.

Virginia, you're not alone in your struggle—and it's by no means a result of your choice to be a vegetarian. Like so many other folks who take various approaches to weight loss (i.e., gluten-free, low-carb, etc.), you are sabotaging your efforts because of your desire to make what you eat succulent, salty, and sweet.

By all means, Virginia, stay true to your convictions and beliefs in your vegetarian lifestyle. But just as you stay true to this lifestyle, stay true to preparing and consuming your foods in their natural state, and minimize the amount of processed breads, supplements, etc. to a bare minimum.

And Virginia, you have to accept that there is more to the fitness spectrum than jogging, as you are breaking down your body parts with this attempt. Find a system that approaches your physical performance with more than just aerobic fitness; a system that implements mobility, corrective exercises, strength, power, and restorative measures.

You'll be hard-pressed to maintain anything other than that slimmer figure you so desire by implementing these changes to your nutrition and performance training. Your beautiful little Vivian will learn lifelong healthy lessons by watching you, and the health of your joints, your emotional state, and ultimately your marriage will appreciate it as well.

AE

CHAPTER 20

Victim Victor

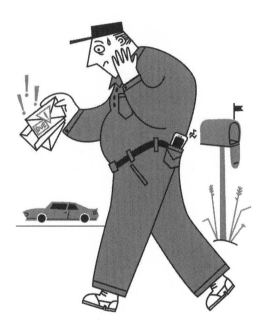

H ardworking Victor, 42, has worked at the same high
school he attended as a student for the past 23 years.
He started working there right after graduation
while attending a local trade school specializing in weld-
ing and carpentry. Young Victor had a great relationship
with the high school principal, as well as the lead custodial
staff, and they were happy to help out the likable 19-year-
old with a part-time janitorial job.

Victor was a go-getter, and it was apparent to those

around him that the instruction he was receiving at the trade school provided a valuable skill set within the school's upkeep and maintenance. Before Victor even completed the interim trade-school program, he found himself working close to a full-time schedule at the school, earning more money than he ever had in his life. With this hard-earned money, Victor financed a brand-new muscle car of his dreams and moved into his own apartment. Victor felt as if he was on cloud nine with his newfound independence.

Once Victor finished with his interim trade school program, he began sending resumes out to various contractors, but received very little response, and those that did respond were offering much lower pay than he was making at the high school. It didn't take long for Victor to see the light and begin full-time status at the high school, where he then entered a union and had a nice little benefits package. A couple of years later, Victor married his high school sweetheart, Veronica.

Today Victor (now 42) and Veronica (now 41) have three children: Vanessa (14), Vera (13), and Victor Jr. (11). Victor serves as the chief custodian at the high school and oversees a staff of seven. Since Victor Jr. started first grade six years ago, Veronica has worked a full-time job as a nurse's aide.

Victor and his family live in a cozy four-bedroom house just outside the city where they grew up, right on the very edge of a large suburban neighborhood. They extended themselves quite a bit on this home, but they loved the location and everything else about it (including the two-and-a-half car garage). Victor has always loved his rides, and he's now on his third dream car, trading up every six to seven years for the newest model, and Veronica has a new, mini SUV.

Starting in the early days of their marriage, Victor and Veronica had a habit of living beyond their means, and that habit continues to this day. They have a premium cable bill in excess of $250 dollars per month, a family plan cell phone bill of over $300 per month (all five of them have smartphones), the two car payments are well over $500 each, and they have an extended home mortgage payment that's been refinanced twice.

Victor and his family also spend quite a bit of money each month on dining out. They stop for fast food three nights a week (and drop a conservative $30–40 for a family of five), and every Saturday they spend at least $100 on a night out at a family style "all-you-can-eat" restaurant for a finer meal.

When Veronica does hit the grocery store, she spends hundreds of dollars on her version of healthy food purchases: multiple boxes of low-fat, honey-coated, sugar-frosted whole grain cereal at over $5 a box; frozen, low-fat waffles at well over $6 a box; lunch meat and tuna salad from the deli at $6-8 per pound; loaves of whole wheat breads; boxes of chewy, chocolate-chip, low-fat granola bars and other "energy" bars; cases of bottled water; yogurt-covered cashews, chocolate-covered raisins, and so on.

This overextension of the family budget has taken a toll on Victor and Veronica's relationship and their personal health. They argue with much bitterness over maxed-out credit cards, various late fees, and finance charges. In addition, Victor, his wife Veronica, and their three children are all overweight. To make matters worse, Victor suffers from many aches and pains, to the point where his manual labor job has become quite the challenge. Ironically, Victor now walks the same hallways where he excelled at multiple sports and didn't have a care or pain in the world when he was a 17-year-old kid.

Veronica's weight gain is the most pronounced, and she takes multiple medications that are a direct result of her excess weight. The irony is not lost on her as she recognizes she is on many if not more of the medications taken by her care patients.

As for the kids, they are unhappy, exasperated, and full of anxiety, particularly on gym days, because they are teased at school about their weight.

Victor's family spends much of their lives in front of the television, on their phones, and on their laptops. Victor blames society in large part for their weight issues, as he feels it's simply too expensive to eat healthy on a combined salary such as theirs, and gym memberships for their entire family are out of reach.

Dear Victor and Veronica,

You are playing the "lower-income victim" by thinking that a healthy lifestyle "rich" in clean and simple foods are out of your financial grasp. What's worse is that you are passing this trait along to your children; as you know, parents lead by example. You are enabling a vicious cycle of food to inflict long-term damage to the health of your family.

Come on, Vic! You're not resorting to fast food every week because it's the most economical choice. You're hitting up your favorite drive-through because it's more convenient, takes less time, and with all the additives, salt, and grease, it just tastes better!

And Veronica, you're not making those grocery store purchases based on finances; you're buying them based on your family's wants (all while the family bank account is being broken).

Victor and Veronica, you're both still young, and your kids' lives are just getting started. Your kids are looking to you both for health and happiness. (Yes, even your teenagers.)

Make changes now. Replace those fast food and all-you-can-eat dinners with healthier and, YES, more economical choices. Pick one day a week (Sunday is ideal) to plan out your menu for the week. Do it together—you'll see; it will bring you closer. Consider buying large portions of economical rice varieties, legumes, potatoes, yams, carrots, greens, and oils (and grab bulk portions of "unprocessed" meats when they are on sale). With regards to the other so-called healthy options Veronica currently makes, purchase large containers of grains such as oats and quinoa to replace those ridiculously priced boxes of cereal; purchase whole grain or sorghum flour and make your own bread and waffles for a fraction of the cost; purchase a few canteens and fill your water from the tap (and save the fate of a few thousand empty plastic bottles from the environment); buy cashews in bulk and forgo the yogurt covering—and as far as the chocolate-covered raisins, chocolate-chip granola bars,

Calling BS, Victor— a healthy lifestyle is not out of your financial grasp.

and energy bars: you guys know better than this!

Victor and Veronica, you also need to alter your material values for the health of your family. Cut back on the cable bill, trade in one of those cars with all the bells and whistles for a cheaper, fuel-economy base model. (Note, Vic: once this last dream car is paid off, no more upgrading; keep it till the wheels fall off). And do your young teens really each need their own smartphone?

Turn your attention to living an active lifestyle and exercising together (you can't afford not to) in place of "expanding" away in front of the television. Build a few garden beds, pick up valuable habits such as canning and freezing your surplus, and put real limits on your family's (and I mean the whole family's) "screen" time (TV, computer, and phone).

Lead, Victor and Veronica, lead...

AE

CHAPTER 21

Doctor Devin

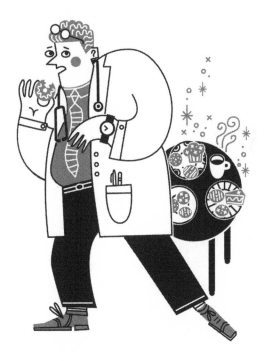

Devin is a prominent primary care specialist who is so highly regarded that he hasn't needed a marketing campaign for new clients in years; they come to him. Essentially, if you don't have a connection to one of his current patients who is willing to pull some strings, there's no chance of getting in with Doc Devin. His nurturing and sincere bedside manner is appreciated by each and every patient, and his intuition along with his knowledge and wisdom seem to allow him to be spot-on in his diagnosis and treatment.

As one would expect of a primary care specialist, Doc Devin obviously deals with a broad array of illnesses and issues, including high blood pressure, high cholesterol, orthopedic injuries, and stress. Interestingly enough, Devin is well aware that many of the illnesses and issues his patients experience are often self-inflicted. He recognizes the poor lifestyle choices that far too many of his patients make, and while he treats many of these issues with medication, he knows that if they would modify their behaviors, so many of their problems could resolve without pills.

Devin puts in long days, as he's truly invested in his work and feels he can make a difference. And as busy as his appointment schedule is, he is a bit of a dinosaur in today's high-stakes medical field, as he will often personally call some of his patients to see how they are feeling and exchange e-mails and texts with them as well.

But aside from Devin's true compassion to heal, Devin works hard filling and surpassing his patient quota for another reason as well. Handsome Doc Devin has earned a handsome six-figure salary for a couple of decades now, and that salary and associated benefits only increase when he's able to see more patients. With his wealth, Devin and his wife, Devlin, have afforded themselves quite an extravagant lifestyle that includes a mini-estate in what's considered the city's best "old money" neighborhood, a condo on the slopes just an hour outside of town, two different social club memberships, matching luxury sedans, and a couple of passports filled with stamps from their many vacations abroad.

Devin spends the day emphasizing to his patients the importance of eating well, exercising, and controlling stress, yet Devin lives somewhat of an unhealthy life that ironically parallels many of his patients. Devin is in his late 40s, and while he's a bigger guy, standing 6'1" tall, he now tips the scales at 250 pounds. His weight has come on slowly over the years, and initially the increasing weight didn't bother him, as he was able to hide it in the office with loose slacks and his doctor's jacket. But his belly can no longer be hidden, and the fat around his neck and face are apparent. Devin knows it and is insecure about it. He also suffers from a significant amount of stress, much of which is related to his workload at his practice. As a result, Devin himself is on a low dose of antidepressants. He has also been experiencing an issue with low sex drive for the past seven years, and even with the recent addition to his personal prescription list—male-enhancing meds—the unwelcome strain on his marriage is palpable.

Notably, Devin's nutrition is a mess. He starts his busy day early with a coffee and croissant as he speeds to the office at six o'clock each morning to read patient files before his appointments begin. When he is able to quickly down lunch in between patients, it usually consists of whatever the nurses are ordering in that day; unfortunately, it's more often than not pizza, hoagies, and dipped and battered Chinese food. To make matters worse, the pharmaceutical reps bring his office doughnuts multiple times each week, and Devin can't help but graze on a couple between his full patient load of upward of 40 patients per day.

On his drive home from the office after gingerly lowering his large frame into his car seat, Devin often finds himself feeling pangs of guilt thinking about what he ate that day. He reflects on his high school and collegiate years. It wasn't that long ago that he was quite the athlete, lettering in three high school sports at a lean 185 pounds and going on to play tennis at a small college before his long, hard-earned journey through medical school.

"Next week, when my schedule lightens, I'll be better about what I eat," he thinks to himself.

From an exercise standpoint, Devin to this day still manages to fit in a quick run on Saturday and Sunday mornings, usually around the neighborhood or the golf course well before the first tee time. However, Devin's knees are bugging him more than ever. Not only does he experience chronic discomfort in his knees from his tennis days, but now jogging with the excess weight has become extremely uncomfortable. Even worse, lately he's been dealing with difficulty walking the stairs and now is dealing with this pain associated with his work as he sits, kneels, and stands with his patients all day.

Devlin is in a similar boat. She, too, was an athlete when she was younger, playing on the women's tennis team at the same college where she met her sweetheart, Devin. Their two lovely children are a bit older, with one in college and one a senior in high school, so now Devlin spends much of her time at the club playing tennis with her friends. Tennis frequently leads to a "quick and casual" lunch with her tennis partner, consisting of maybe a club sandwich with fries, or a gourmet club half-pound burger on the club's famous brioche bun. Lunch almost always includes a glass of wine—and a glass of wine often turns into another glass of wine. Aside from tennis and a morning walk with their two pedigreed pooches, Devlin also trains with a group of friends one time each week with the club's Director of Personal Training.

Devlin is 5'7" tall, and although she was a lean 130 pounds in her college tennis days, she now tips the scale at 180 pounds. She is quite unhappy with her appearance, experiencing more aches and pains, often feeling tired throughout the day, and also suffering from occasional depression, for which Devin prescribed her a low dose of antidepressants. Devlin doesn't feel sexually appealing any longer, and one can only guess it's due to a combination of her appearance and her insecurities regarding Devin's sexual issues. Her lack of mobility, particularly on the tennis court, frustrates her. But she enjoys her spoiled lifestyle, and disguises much of her unhappiness by purchasing custom-fitted clothes that hide much of her added weight.

In the evenings following long, stressful days at the office, Devin and Devlin have dinner together at one of their clubs at least two or three times each week. Their high school daughter is generally off on her own, now, with evening practices or spending time with her own friends. Unfortunately, Devin and Devlin do not make the best choices at the club's restaurant, and usually have a cocktail or two as well. They also frequently dine out on the weekends at both of their favorite Italian and steak house restaurants, often meeting up with another couple or two and enjoying an extended evening of finer foods and wines.

From an outside perspective, Devin seems to have it all: a rewarding, lucrative career, a great family, a huge home and condo in the mountains, luxury cars, prestigious club memberships, travel, many evenings out at the city's finer establishments, and more. Yet he's struggling with huge amounts of stress on a daily basis, his body and joints are breaking down, and he and his wife are both overweight and their sex life is in need of resuscitation. And then there's the nagging guilt of hypocrisy which he suppresses by rationalizing a too-busy work schedule that weighs heavily on his mind—and body.

How can he continue to preach wellness, yet look and feel like "hell-ness?"

Dear Devin,

It's hard to comprehend the irony of spending your day preaching healthy lifestyles, yet both you and your wife struggle to implement these same behaviors. This is such compelling insight into just how much of a role the lure of food (salty, succulent, and sweet) and quest for material acquisitions play in our lives. If so many of the most rigorously trained health professionals struggle (and they do), then light should clearly be shed on the challenges we all face.

Oh, the irony of spending your day preaching healthy lifestyles, when you struggle to implement these same behaviors.

Devin and Devlin, you both need to prioritize the health of your bodies and minds. We only get one body and one mind—there are no do-overs.

Step away from the manufactured world of material attainment and retention you've put yourselves in and focus on simplifying your lives. You've raised two beautiful children, but your impact on them is not even close to being over. Eat out less. Spend time shopping and preparing meals together. Begin a sensible and sustainable training program. Consider a hobby where you can tend to a small garden of fresh herbs and veggies, and possibly downsize some of the "material" in your life so you can cut down on your patient load, and as a result, much of your stress.

And pass on this newfound humility to your girls.

You two have many zestful, intimate decades ahead of you if you can find balance and humility. AGE well Devin and Devlin—AGE with grace...

AE

CHAPTER 22

Jet-Setting Jack

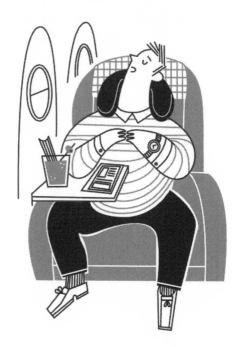

Jack sits at the men's-only bar of his posh country club, his fifth vodka tonic in hand, slurring his sob story to any of his golfing buddies who stick around to listen. Last night, Jack discovered a salacious e-mail thread between his wife and another man. And to top off that punch-in-the-gut revelation, his morning began with an explosive argument with his kids, who called him out for being their "missing in action" dad. Jack is stunned that his perfect life is crumbling before his eyes.

Jack grew up in what many would call a privileged manner. He and his older brother Jake attended private schools, received brand new cars at 16, and never worked as teenagers because their parents wanted them to focus on lacrosse and academics. Jack and Jake lived similar lives after high school as they attended a private college where their tuition, room and board, and living expenses were fully covered by their parents.

Now in his late 30s, Jack has done very well for himself running a third-generation construction company where Jake is Vice President of Operations. Jack has managed to maintain much of the midsize business of close to 80 employees that his grandfather established in 1964. However, his abrasive and absentee management style during his short tenure has led to quite a bit of key employee turnover.

Jack is married to Jennifer, and they have two kids. They live in a wealthy neighborhood in the suburbs, their kids go to private schools, they have a nanny, the highest-end SUV, a limited-edition foreign sedan, and Jack has his beloved convertible two-seater. They are also members of an exclusive country club as well as a prestigious social club in the area.

Jack is involved with a couple of elite young executive peer groups that travel numerous times each year to meet up at lavish resorts for brainstorming, strategic planning, and—of course—networking. Jack and his executive buddies have traveled as far as New Zealand and China for week-long retreats in order to collaborate on and negotiate big-time deals.

While traveling, Jack flies first class and likes to be served his cocktails and hors d'oeuvres during the flight.

He only dines at the finest steak, seafood, French, and Italian restaurants in the world, where the highest-priced wines and premium fare are on the menu.

While he's away, Jack occasionally gets an executive-style workout in at his resort, where he hits some light cardio on the elliptical while reading the latest business news, then takes a nice long steam. This complements his routine when he's at home, where he performs his circuit workout with a personal trainer at his country club.

In addition to insisting on having the finer things in life, Jack likes to be part of the "in" crowd. He attends most of the big events, like Super Bowls, the World Series, and the hottest concerts—almost always with VIP status. Jack doesn't refrain from letting you know about the famous people he knows and hangs out with as a member of the "in" crowd. He also doesn't shy away from letting you know the places he's been and all of the "top" things he's accomplished. Essentially, Jack knows how to talk about Jack.

However, Jack also misses most of his kids' events: their first games, concerts, science fairs, and more, as he's extremely busy "working the deal." Jack has never even considered coaching one of his children's sports teams and has no time to help with homework or study with his kids.

As far as Jack's health is concerned, his recent physical for an increased life insurance policy revealed that he's prediabetic, moderately obese, and has high cholesterol. Since Jack knows his insurance guy well and spends a lot of money with him, some strings are pulled to make sure Jack gets his increased policy.

At first glance, Jack seems to have it all: he's a young, wealthy guy with the perfect family and has all the lavish materials at his fingertips. But behind the facade, he has kids who resent him and are now rebelling in ways that are soon to manifest themselves, a wife that is considering an affair with an old male "friend" with whom she's reconnected on social media, and his own personal health is in disarray. As for his actual facade, Jack is sporting a one-inch layer of fat that seems to cover most of his body, including his face, neck, chest, stomach, legs, and even his ankles.

Dear Jack,

You're being a jackass. You are oblivious to the fact that you are paying a dire price for all of your so-called professional and material successes. You have a boatload of cash and travel like a prima donna, yet your wife is on the verge of having a physical affair with a man who ironically couldn't put a dent into your earnings. Your kids look up to their teachers and their coaches more than they do their father, and your own body and health are a mess.

Jack, you're so caught up in "Jack" that what is really important has taken an economy-row seat.

Jack, you're so caught up in "Jack" that what is really important has taken an economy-row seat. Quite frankly, things are only going to get worse unless you take a really hard look at your bloated, egotistical self in the mirror. No matter your material conquests, you can't buy family happiness, nor can you simply throw money at your own health to look and feel better. Holy hell, man, even when you cry "woe is me," you do it at the men's-only bar at your country club.

Screw the braggadocious Super Bowls, World Series, etc., and get involved as an assistant coach on your kids' sports teams. Find out what makes your wife happy, because clearly it's not the money. Begin to lead your family—and your company, for that matter—from a more grounded approach. Take care of your own health, physique, and physical performance through proper training and nutrition, and let your healthy lifestyle serve as an example to your family as well as your company. Help change the health of others around you Jack—be a true leader!

Come off that pompous high horse you're on and seek humility.

AE

CHAPTER 23

Trucker Trey

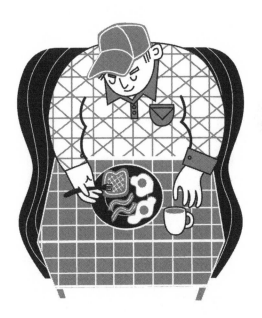

T rey is quite the monster of a man. He stands 6′5″ tall, and to this day he still carries around his imposing figure the way he did throughout his sporting years of high school and college, although he's now about 100 pounds heavier than his playing days. Trey starred in both football and basketball in high school, where he was an all-state selection for both sports in his junior and senior seasons and went on to excel at basketball for two years on a scholarship to a Division 2 school in his home state.

Playing at the Division 2 level was competitive and gave Trey the challenges and successes he had become so accustomed to since his early teenage years. But Trey soon realized that being a college athlete required a massive amount of commitment beyond his already challenging basic studies. So after two years of what Trey felt like was a grind, not to mention quite a bit of wear and tear on his knees, Trey came to the realization that playing at the Division 2 level was never going to get him a shot in the pros, and he decided that college was not for him.

When Trey stepped away from campus life, he was 20 years old. It wasn't long before his parents began pushing him to land a permanent job and consider moving out of their house. Trey knew they were right and knew he had to get himself out of his "I left college, now what do I do?" slump. He was able to pick up a full-time job working the nighttime shift at the loading docks for a large warehouse. Before long, Trey was doing well, making a $35K a year salary with the ability to crack $40K with some overtime.

Trey discovered he was a bit of a celebrity among his coworkers on the docks, as his athletic superstar reputation from his high school days preceded him. And with his 6'5", 250-pound frame, though 25 pounds heavier than his playing days, he appeared to be full of what seemed like even more muscle, which continued to add to his lure.

The warehouse manager was a huge sports fan and had always liked Trey. So after two years of watching Trey working diligently on the loading docks, he took Trey aside and suggested he consider entering their Commercial Driver's License program, where he could learn to operate a tractor trailer and increase his earning potential significantly and put a little less manual wear on his body.

Before long Trey was driving a big rig, living on a bigger salary, living in a bigger apartment, and becoming much bigger in physical status as well.

Trey had always liked to eat, and back in high school and college and even during his two years on the loading docks, Trey was so active and genetically gifted (and had youth on his side), that he could pretty much eat whatever he wanted and maintain his large, muscular physique. But the trucking lifestyle traditions that unfortunately so often catch up to drivers began to catch up with Trey as well.

Trey's eight-to-ten-hour shifts on the road include frequent rest stops for fuel, and ultimately the opportunity for fast food, loaded coffees, and snacks like soda, chips, and candy bars from the gas station convenience stores or vending machines. Trey sleeps in his rig quite often before his turnaround, so he generally keeps a supply of food for breakfasts, lunches, dinners, and snacks inside the rig. His stash includes ample quantities of quick-grab salty and sweet munchies, as well as the leftover containers of food he orders at the trucker-friendly diners, like biscuits and gravy, pancakes and bacon, meatloaf, mashed potatoes with more gravy, and a bunch of buttered dinner rolls. And of course, he keeps his trusty thermos filled with "high octane" coffee, as he likes to call it.

At 33 years old, Trey weighs in at a whopping 330 pounds and is on medication for both his Type 2 diabetes and his high blood pressure. Trey's son Troy, who is an 11-year-old hoop star in the 5th grade, worships his dad and everything he's taught him about the game of basketball. Sadly, Trey can no longer play much more than a basic game of shoot around H-O-R-S-E with his boy. He's out of shape as he performs zero exercise, and his knees absolutely ache from the long hauls and the 100-plus pounds of added weight he carries around on his machine. And Trey's high school sweetheart and now wife of 11 years, Tia, has also put on a significant amount of weight, following many of the same eating habits as Trey, and she, too, is experiencing lifestyle-related health issues as well as image issues.

Dear Trey,

Man, you need to look at what you're doing to yourself and your family. You are 33 years old, and with your habits, you may never be around to see Troy play his senior season in high school. You are providing for your family, but the decline in your health is far outweighing what you're earning.

Did I mention you were only 33 years old?

Dang man, you should still be out there posting up against your little guy, playing him one-on-one, training with him, and eating healthy with him. You're living like an old man beyond your years. Trey, you need to lead your son by example.

And Trey, don't dare blame the trucker lifestyle for your condition. You make choices to eat this way because you, like so many, desire the salty, savory, and sweet you get from the garbage you're eating.

Eating garbage is not a mandatory requirement for big-rig drivers. You could easily pack your cooler with fruits such as apples, bananas, oranges, and pears, and consume those with a small handful of nuts that you packed in bulk (which would easily replace those candy bars). And rather than the chips you think you need to snack on, how about a large container of cut-up carrots, celery, tomato, and sugar snap peas, along with some homemade guacamole (i.e., smashed avocado and sea salt). And what's with all those breakfasts and dinners at the diner, Trey? Pack some hard-boiled eggs, some Greek yogurt, berries, and cooked oats for breakfast, and a large tossed salad with grilled chicken and quinoa, and eat like the athlete that you still can be. By the way Trey, you'll save a boatload of money this way as well!

...don't dare blame the trucker lifestyle for your condition.

Yes, Trey, a career in hauling can have its lonely moments, but not only do you make a good living, you're able to be around on the weekends and some evenings with your family. Use this time to transform the way you approach food and begin to exercise intelligently. Your son Troy idolizes you, and you have your high school sweetheart at your side. Help guide your family to a happy, healthy lifestyle. Eat what can be fished, grown, and butchered, begin a sustainable training program for you and Tia and a touch more detailed training for Troy by way of properly programmed sports performance training. Skip those trips to the diner and get back home sooner, man.

It's time to turn back the clock and live like the 6'5", 225-pound stud you are under that 330-pound facade. We all have our temptations, our cultures, and our stressors, but no matter these challenges, we must humble ourselves to Mother Nature, Trey.

AE

CHAPTER 24

Not-So-Humble Heath

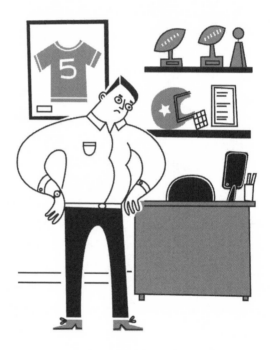

Heath, who recently received a master's degree in sports medicine, can't believe his luck. At 24 he was selected from a large pool of qualified candidates for what promised to be his dream job. His hometown's professional football team hired Heath to work alongside the athletes as part of the team's sports medicine staff. For Heath, landing the position felt like karma. Having excelled at college football at an academically driven university as an undergrad, it was starting to look as though he may get invited to some local pro days to showcase his skills, until an injury in his senior year put the brakes on that dream. It was that twist of fate, along with encouragement from his girlfriend, Hannah, that convinced Heath to pursue his master's degree, which consequently landed him a job that immersed him in the sport he loved.

Right out of the gate as a junior member of the sports medicine staff, Heath worked closely with the physicians and coaches to provide the athletes with therapeutic screening, support, monitoring, and return-to-play strategies that put his education as well as his love for the sport to good use. Heath was smart, dedicated, and had a humble work ethic, something that made him stand out among the other twentysomethings on the staff.

But to Heath, the most satisfying and motivating aspect of his work was seeing his rehabilitation efforts with the athletes make a difference in their long-term health. He spent many of his off-hours continuing to educate himself on the current research findings and therapies in his field of sports medicine. He took the initiative to develop individual training programs for athletes to help prevent injuries. The players and coaches admired and appreciated Heath's efforts and know-how.

Not too long into his career, the senior staff and coaches along with the team's owners took note of the efforts and hard work of this talented young man.

Heath loved his day-to-day work helping and healing athletes. But the job had another notable aspect that really appealed to him as well: he was around money—LOTS of money—and lots of people who made lots of money.

As a kid, Heath grew up with much less than most of

the other kids in his school district, which was one of the wealthier districts in the area. He realized early on that his parents were not able to provide him with the high-end bikes, toys, and video game systems that other kids in his elementary school owned. While other kids at his school told stories about their family summer vacations to the islands and abroad, Heath rarely talked about how he spent most of his summers working on his aunt's and uncle's farm. To a young kid, having to get up at the crack of dawn to tend to livestock and crops and working afternoons at their roadside market didn't seem like something to brag about to his buddies.

By high school, he envied the kids who showed up each year with new, brand-name sneakers. A combined athletic and academic scholarship paid Heath's way to a prestigious university, where he was struck by the number of students with new cars and high-end apartments, paid in full by their parents.

His humble upbringing pitted against the affluence that surrounded him weighed heavily on young Heath. As a teen, he had made a promise to himself he would one day live a life of wealth, where he could provide his one-day family with anything they wanted.

As young Heath's career continued to soar, so did his lifestyle. Because he was so well liked and respected by so many higher-ups in the ball club, Heath soon found himself being invited to spend time outside of work with those in power—not just within the organization, but also those connected to professional sports: CEOs, politicians, celebrities, investors, and other "luxury boxers," as Heath privately called them.

By the time he was 28, the team's ownership recognized Heath's knowledge of the game, work ethic, and charm, and felt that his talents would best serve the Front Office working for the club's vice president. With that came a hefty salary promotion. And while Heath knew the job meant leaving behind the work he loved, the compensation and benefits were calling his name, and he knew he would be on his way to accumulating the material things he had always wanted.

A couple of years later, Heath's new career and new-found friendships among the wealthy elite had him living a very new lifestyle. He played golf at prestigious private clubs, ate at premier restaurants, and bought custom-tailored clothes. He purchased a one-bedroom condo with an amazing view of the city's sports arena and the best sports car his paycheck could afford him.

Heath's life was a far cry from what he knew growing up. He had everything he had set his sights on. His life goals were fulfilled, and yet 30-year-old Heath was not.

For the first time in his life, Heath did not like who he saw in the mirror, both literally and figuratively. Heath didn't like that his face looked red and somewhat bloated, his belly was beginning to hang over his midline, and his once-firm chest muscles had become, well, not so firm. His late nights at the office, business travel, and social obligations barely left time for workouts. He rarely thought about nutrition since choosing off the menu at a high-end restaurant or from room service was his new normal.

And he was tired. The travel involved with his new job, as well as the thoughts of his daunting mortgage and car payments, seemed to disrupt his sleep. He rarely got more than four or five hours a night. Ironically, the business travel also meant he barely spent time in the condo or drove his new car.

And he was lonely. His relationship with his college sweetheart, Hannah, who was working as a special-needs teacher in their hometown, had been over for a couple of years. Heath's focus on conquering "material," not to mention the constant travel, put a not-unexpected strain on this once like-minded couple.

The so-called friendships Heath had developed over the past few years were more like business relationships. And he started to see that many of the people he was socializing and doing business with were unhappy too. No matter how much wealth they accumulated, it couldn't mask the obvious. Their health was in disarray, their bodies looked like hell, many were in poor or split marriages, and sadly, many of their kids weren't speaking to them.

Sitting alone in his first-class seat on a cross-country trip and staring down at the letter in his hand offering him a new job as vice president of a major ball club in a city on the other side of the country left Heath feeling lost. Sick, even. Unsure what to do.

He folded the letter. As he gazed out the plane's window, he could see nothing but vast farmlands below. He wondered what life was like for those farmers as he remembered fondly his summers on the farm and the lessons they taught him.

He wondered what he should do, and he wondered about the one person who would know what he should do: Hannah.

Dear Heath,

You're at a major crossroads in your life, and most of us have been there. I've been there. But you need to get the hell away from there.

Heath, stop. Step back to truly examine your day to day. Really take a look at what your life has become—at who you're answering to and what your focus has become. You worked hard to land a dream job so that you could use your knowledge and love of a discipline to help and heal people. And you took pride in it, you were good at it, and you made a difference.

You also took pride in yourself— your health and appearance. Now you feel and kind of look like crap.

Dude, WTF?

You look and feel like crap.

Dude, WTF?

And then there's Hannah. She was the one who kept you grounded and humble; who shared your dreams of a simple, comfortable life—one with children and faith.

Heath, you're still a young guy with a long life ahead of you. Take what you've learned, not just from the profession you love, but from what you don't love about the life you have made and those whose lives you've seen.

You need to make the right choices before it's too late. Reinvent yourself back to who you used to be, and go back to making a real difference, not just making real money.

And by the way, I've heard Hannah isn't seeing anyone right now. Don't be an ass. Don't let her get away again.

AE

CHAPTER 25

Happy-Healthy-Humble Heath

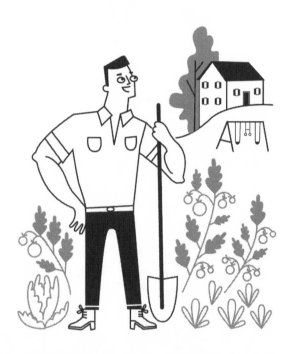

Author's Note: I couldn't bring this book to a close without writing a sweet ending for at least one of my characters. Hence, Not-So-Humble Heath makes life choices that transform him into Happy-Healthy-Humble Heath.

Heath and Hannah now live in a small home on a modest piece of land. They've built a large garden, added a few chickens, and have spent valuable time together learning the ins and outs of sustainability. Heath's sports car is a thing of the past. He's driving a small 4x4 pickup that serves a functional purpose for their garden life.

Heath and Hannah's life together took on wonderful new meaning when they had two beautiful children (Heath Jr. and Haley), and they took pride in raising them in a modest, faith-filled lifestyle. Heath and Hannah sent their kids to school with a home-cooked meal full of fruits and veggies, and have kept the amount of school lunches of pizza and fried chicken to a minimum. They kept ice cream after the ball game to be a special occasion rather than the norm. They limited their kids' time in front of the television, did not provide them with cell phones, and taught their children basic chores at a young age. They introduced them to the garden, allowed them to get their hands dirty, encouraged them to play outside every day, raised them to be respectful and thankful, and infused them with the importance of giving back.

> Not-So-Humble Heath makes life choices that transform him into Happy-Healthy-Humble Heath.

Hannah continues to work part-time with special-needs kids, and Heath started his own sports medicine clinic where he works with middle school, high school, and college athletes, as well as older adults. While he's devoted to his work, he made a decision early on to not overextend himself to try to grow the business to multiple locations. His focus is on his family and providing for them, but providing in a way that allows him to be part of it, not apart from it. Heath surrounded himself with a like-minded, hardworking staff who he relies on and trusts to handle things when he can't be there.

Heath's and Hannah's marriage grew stronger each year. They shared the same values when it came to raising Heath Jr. and Haley, they prepared and cooked healthy meals together, they both made time to train regularly (and sensibly) to help keep their bodies lean, strong, and supple, they practiced their faith as a family, and they valued that which was truly valuable—rather than material things. Their commitment to each other (and to their healthy bodies) seemed to have an added benefit—a kickass love life.

Hey, what can I say? I'm a hopeless romantic.

Tough Love For The Masses

(A THREE-STEP PLAN)

In the Welcome Letter, I asked you to put aside any preconceived notions and boiling tempers during the read. This book was not written to be purposely offensive, ignorant, cruel, or to embarrass anyone in any way. On the contrary, *Tough Love Letters* drills somewhat deeply into these characters' fat, unfit, unhealthy, and unhappy lives with sincerity and purpose. It was done with the intention that you or your spouse, family members, or significant other may connect to one or a combination of these characters to shed light on the problems we all face and to ultimately elicit change.

Now that you've had a chance to get to know the cast of characters, their struggles, and my letters to them, let's ask ourselves a few questions: Are we conquering all of our financial and material desires? Are we living our lives idolizing others? Are we living a life of gluttonous food behaviors? And as a result, have we compromised too much in the process? Has our general health been violated? Do we no longer find ourselves sexually attractive? Have our relationships with our family been breached? Do we move through life fatigued, stressed, deconditioned, injury-prone, sad, and miserable?

If the answer is "yes" to any of these questions, you know in your heart that it's time for **change**.

But let me be very clear: I am not defining "change" as a journey toward a fitness-pageant-perfect body or performing as an Olympic-level athlete. Nor am I suggesting completely giving up on all the foods that we enjoy. (Life without ice cream every so often is really not worth living, in my opinion.)

However, we must find some middle ground here. The majority of us are excessively fat (yes, I used the F-word again), very unfit, have a multitude of self-inflicted health issues, and are unhappy.

Our struggles are real and challenging. And I get that it's painful. I get that it's crazy difficult to gain control. Almost everyone struggles! Personal trainers struggle (yes, even personal trainers), sports coaches struggle, doctors struggle, nutritionists struggle, life coaches struggle, attorneys struggle, police officers struggle, stay-at-home moms and dads struggle, teachers struggle, nurses struggle, business owners struggle. I struggle. There are very few people who do not struggle.

But there is hope! Just as I laid out specific calls to action for each of my characters, I am proposing a **Three-Step Tough Love Plan of Action** for you, my reader.

1. Get Your F*cking Priorities in Line

(Forgive me, sort of, for my last piece of much-emphasized, yet appropriate allusion to profanity.) We're stressed to unprecedented levels trying to live far beyond necessary means in our thirst to attain material possessions. The newest smartphones, the latest fashions, luxury cars, the largest flat-screens, the premium cable plans, or the biggest homes have become our focus. We're wasting our lives on social media, being overly fascinated with the lives of others—those we know and those we want to know, like celebrities. Oh, and then there's our preoccupation with professional sports and athletes (my personal pet peeve). We watch hours of TV, with hundreds of digital or satellite premier sport-package stations to scroll through, or we attend sporting events season after season, basically living our lives idolizing others while in spectator mode. Why? Why do we spend more time with our butts on the couch or in stadium seats than we do with our butts in the game?

You absolutely need to step off the connectivity grid for a period to reflect on your life's purpose without the noise and multitude of stressors. Shut the phone down for a couple of days. Unplug the laptop. Throw the remotes in a drawer. The world will continue to turn, and you will survive this epic sacrifice! Escape for a couple of days to a mountain retreat, lakeside cabin, or beach. (This does not need to be the Taj Mahal of resorts, but can be something much more simple and basic.) You need to be able to think clearly and rationally and leave the daily grind of excess earnings, the quest for material goods, the constant connectivity to social media, and the idolization of others behind you. Use this time to evaluate your finances, your acquisitions, and your ego, and then put priorities in place. Figure out your purpose.

2. Jump on the ALLTRAIN (alltrainllc.com)

You need a lifelong plan to strategic, safe, and sustainable physical fitness and performance training. You can no longer fool yourselves into thinking that joining a $5/month, 24/7 fitness center to join thousands of other hamsters on wheels will solve your deeply ingrained issues. Nor are the high-intensity, balls-to-the-wall group classes going to offer you anything other than the likelihood of eventual injury and dysfunction. (You're no spring chicken!) And picking up the long-distance running option is a one-dimensional approach, and worse, will most likely break down your lean mass, your joints, and ultimately your will.

ALLTRAIN will eliminate the plethora of fitness fuss that surrounds you and will help you become a leaner, stronger, more functional and powerful being. You will no longer be injury-prone or vulnerable, but on the contrary, you will be built to compete in the sport of everyday life. You will be well prepared to play with your kids or grandkids with zest, work vigorously in the yard, tackle small home remodel projects with confidence, or even play a recreational sport.

With ALLTRAIN, you may crawl, jump, leap, throw, roll, twist, rotate, extend, and flex. You may swing kettlebells, press dumbbells, pull on bands, don a weighted vest, battle a rope, or lug a sandbag. But here's the big catch: you'll do this with purpose in mind, not just because it sounds cool. You will not do things irrationally or incompetently. ALLTRAIN's strategic, safe, and sustainable programming will provide you with a clear-cut, long-term plan that will transcend the demands of life's varying terrains with vigor and surety.

3. Embrace PLAIN Nutrition (alltrainllc.com/plain)

You need a precise plan to a plain and simple, lifelong approach to food. Today's masses are eerily similar to herds of cattle vying for a spot at the grain troughs. Whether we wait in line for the famous cheese dogs, waffle cones, or funnel cakes at the amusement park or boardwalk; or we form a mad dash to the food court at the airport before our next ninety-minute flight; or we idle impatiently at the drive-through to satisfy our insatiable hunger for fast food favorites, we emulate these cattle herds.

And the rationalized, half-assed approaches we take with low-carb, high-protein, low-fat, fasting, gluten-free, grass-fed, vegan, organic, non-GMO, calorie-tapering diets and more in an attempt to counter our struggles are virtually ineffective.

The PLAIN Nutrition program will eradicate the nutrition noise that besieges you and will guide you to becoming a leaner, healthier, happier human being.

Tough Love Parting Thoughts

Dear Reader,

It is time to get your groove back. If your body is a wreck due to excessive endurance training, high-intensity training, or simply zero training, you're fat as f*ck (I fibbed a little; I used the F-bomb and alluded to the real F-BOMB one last time), you're on a bunch of medications related directly to a poor lifestyle, and you're unhappy—change it. Don't settle for mediocrity or what has become the sedentary norm.

A growing number of 30-, 40-, 50-, 60-, and 70-plus-year-olds (real people) are adhering to my **Three-Step Tough Love Plan of Action** and are whipping your ass in the game of life. That's right, 30-year-olds finding out they can sprint without injury, 40-year-olds discovering more strength than they had in their teens and twenties, 50-year-olds more supple than kids half their age, 60-year-olds capable of jumping over a three-foot hurdle without injury, 70-year-olds performing pushups with a thirty-pound vest on their back (and I'm talking full range, chest to the floor, no droopy-rear-end pushups), and don't think I'm alienating the 80-year-old club, as I've seen firsthand these warriors maintain a level of strength, power, and vigor well beyond many twenty to thirty years younger—and they are all lean machines, primarily consuming foods that can be fished, grown, or butchered. All the while they continue the fight to keep life's priorities in check.

I truly hope *Tough Love Letters* helps you find purpose beyond material quests, food seduction, and living life through others and you begin to take pride in your body and your being.

Sincerely,
Albert Eiler

Appendix: Just a Few More...

....

While each of my 25 star-studded cast members depicts so many of the Fat, Unfit, Unhealthy, and Unhappy of our society, there are other folks I've met along the way (or not... I'll never tell) who I just can't ignore, but didn't make the 25-character final cut. (What can I say? They didn't audition well.) They, like the others, have ventured down a path of wrong or wandering choices that resulted in woes, weight gain, and not-so-wellness.

Fasting Freddy – proudly touts to all when he's on one of his various "disciplined" fasting regimens, such as a 36-hour dry fast, a 24-hour water fast, or a daily 18-hour intermittent fast. He actually drops 10-25 pounds with each short term attempt (a portion of this is lean muscle), but then gains back all the weight (but with no lean muscle) after his sacrificial moments have expired and he enters his post-fast gorging frenzy.

Tribal-Diet Troy – believes foraging, fishing and functional movement like his "ancestors" did is the path to fantastic health. Yet Troy's body is an injury-laden wreck from excessive amounts of "functional" exercise...and he's 30 pounds overweight to boot. Apparently, his ancestors also liked fast food.

Neo Ned – boasts that he's tried the latest, most advanced, hottest fitness and wellness trends: cryotherapy, lava rock massages, oxygen chambers, infrared saunas—not to mention his bootcamp-style training with ex-US military special forces. He even ships in grass-fed bison from the Midwest, special berries from the Himalayas, and root vegetables from South America to impress his dinner guests. Yet despite his love for what's hot, he ignores what he's got: nagging injuries from one too many soldier-like wall climbs, a definite double chin, and a belly that hangs well over his manhood. It seems the idea of strategic, safe, and sustainable training along with nutrition done plain and simple utterly bore his neonarcissist nature.

Nurse Nancy – works a challenging evening work schedule of two consecutive 12-hour shifts, followed by two days off, then repeats. The overtime she earns comes in very handy with the large mortgage and car payments she and her hubby Nick face, as well as the kids' music lessons, camps, clinics, phones, satellite packages, and food bills. Nancy's work highlights are the delivery meal she and her peers will decide on and pitch in for at their extended break, ranging from pizza to hoagies to calzones to burgers and fries. Nancy also enjoys two 15-minute breaks during her shift, where she attacks the vending machine for a soda and either chips or a candy bar. Nancy is 60 pounds overweight, but even more concerning is the fact that Nancy is on both blood pressure and cholesterol meds, has chronic fatigue, is extremely unhappy with her appearance, and is heading into a depressive state. Sadly, Nancy is becoming the patient she has honorably cared for over countless years.

Personal Trainer Pete – with his master's degree in kinesiology, Pete is a big fish in a small pond, since most of his fellow "trainers" at the boutique health club where he works are not fitness specialists, but more closely resemble a team of front desk, administrative, and floor attendants. Pete holds the title of Head Trainer and is responsible for programming the weekly workouts as well as designing specialized diet strategies for VIP clients that include: cutting carbs, fasting, increasing protein, using supplements, calorie tapering, and more. But ironically, Pete is a big fish for other reasons: he has quite the noticeable belly on his beefy frame and very little definition to the rest of his body. It seems that while he dutifully packs a healthy workday lunch to lead by example, single-dude-living-alone Pete likes to knock down a few beers and a dozen wings most evenings, and can't pass on the extra helpings of pasta and garlic toast at Nana's Sunday dinners.

Millennial Molly – never worked much during high school and college, aside from some minor volunteer positions for camps and clinics. While in college, she racked up quite the student loan total, using these funds to cover her education as well as room, board, books, meals, clothing, laptop, printer, and of course a smartphone. Come career-search time, her resume looked solid from an educational standpoint, but revealed very little work experience, and she hasn't interviewed very well (particularly when she continues to look at her cell phone during the interview process). Her sheltered life has her in quite the bubble, where she thinks chicken and fish are raised at the grocery store, and water comes from a bottle. (While this is a bit of an exaggeration, the point is she doesn't have much of a clue about real life.) What is more, Molly is 25 pounds overweight because she is used to eating what she wants, when she wants; her relationships are shallow via dating apps, and she is struggling with anxiety over her career search.

Organic Omar – a "huge" health-conscious guy who drives across town to shop at the premier organic grocery, purchasing everything from organic berries and veggies to non-GMO grains, meats, and wild-caught fish. He even purchases his soaps, lotions, and toothpaste at the organic grocery. He hits a trendy yoga studio three times per week, twisting and turning in a 100-degree room while sweating profusely ("cleansing," as he sees it). Omar also likes to hit the sustainably produced IPA brewery pretty hard, as well as the clean and green cabernets at the local winery with his other organically minded friends. Alas, even with his organically driven life, Omar is 20 pounds overweight, feels as though he lacks sufficient strength and power, and is a bit bummed.

Gut Health Gus – can't talk enough about or get enough "healthy" bacteria in his microbiome, stocking up on supplements and superfoods. (Kefir and yogurts are a daily must, and a variety of gut cleansing teas fill his refrigerator.) Still, he often munches on frozen toaster-oven pizzas, chips, and diet sodas in the late evening as he watches his prime time sports.

Wino Wally – walks five miles most days to stay fit and does his best to eat a strict, mostly plant-based dinner each night. Wally proudly pairs most meals with an expensive bottle of red from his cellar. After all, if wine is high in anti-oxidants, a more expensive vintage must have even more of these disease-fighting agents. Nonetheless, Wally is puzzled by the fact that despite his "healthy, high-end habits," he's 15 pounds overweight and has very little muscle mass on his body, to the point that he's soft and mushy...not unlike grapes that have fallen off the vine.

Life Coach Lexi – has a handful of clients, mostly married women, with whom she lays out a very matter of fact, strong-willed course of self-improvement and empowerment. Ironically, Lexi herself is in a mess of a marriage, where her husband has stepped out on her with one of her closest friends (she was a bit lax in following her own coaching advice and forgot to pay attention to Lex); she is fighting an excess of 35 pounds that comes in the shape of a pear; and under her secure portrayal is a very insecure, emotionally distraught woman who also struggles with her diet, particularly her pattern of finding comfort in food.

Infomercial Ida – it's 1:00 a.m., and she's channel surfing the tube, where a 30-minute ad for the latest butt-lifting DVD is on. "Knowing" this is the answer to her weight issue (just like the ab-crunching device or the pound-shredding pills that preceded it), she snags her smartphone from her nightstand and places her order before she drifts off to sleep. The package arrives 4–5 days later and sits unopened in her foyer for 4–5 months until she decides it would make a good donation to her church's rummage sale.

Prepackaged-Meal-Plan Peggy – eats most of her meals from "tasty," microwaveable packages delivered monthly (lasagna, meatloaf, spaghetti and meatballs, pot pies, and more...all at only 300 calories each.) Oh, and she decides to stop exercising because her daily calorie count might be too low to sustain her through her workouts. She loses weight quickly (including muscle) but then gains all the fat back (and then some) once the pricey monthly plan proceeds to pummel her pocketbook.

Sabotage Sue – enthusiastically commits to a clean-eating plan for a few weeks at a time and sees some nice progress toward her weight-loss goals. But then her deadline-driven working-mom schedule, her can't-miss-one social (read: "cocktail-heavy") commitment and, for that matter, her no-denying-it, lazy sweet tooth all provide convenient excuses to stray from her steadfastness, thus sabotaging her successes, and soon she's back to square one.

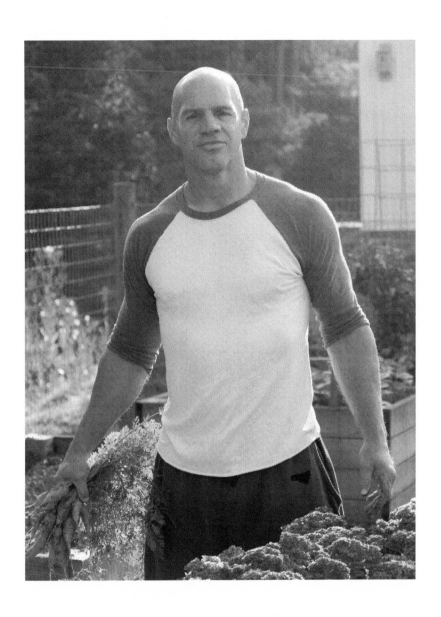

ALBERT EILER

Made in the USA
Middletown, DE
08 February 2020